NO WHINING

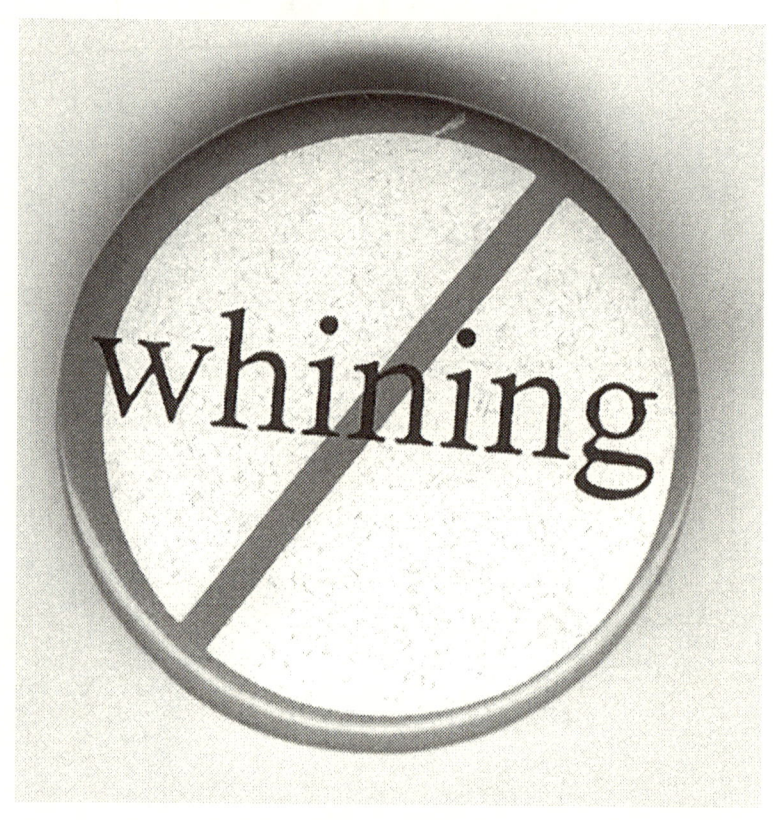

Other iUniverse books by Herb Tabak

Wheres the Runway? And Other Flying Stories

Colorado High Country Anthology

NO WHINING

✦

Craig Hospital Spinal Injury Rehab: Reaching New Heights

Herb Tabak

Edited by Faye Quam Heimerl

iUniverse, Inc.

New York Lincoln Shanghai

NO WHINING
Craig Hospital Spinal Injury Rehab: Reaching New Heights

iUniverse books may be ordered through booksellers or by contacting:

iUniverse
2021 Pine Lake Road, Suite 100
Lincoln, NE 68512
www.iuniverse.com
1-800-Authors (1-800-288-4677)

ISBN-13: 978-0-595-37814-2 (pbk)
ISBN-13: 978-0-595-67567-8 (cloth)
ISBN-13: 978-0-595-82193-8 (ebk)
ISBN-10: 0-595-37814-5 (pbk)
ISBN-10: 0-595-67567-0 (cloth)
ISBN-10: 0-595-82193-6 (ebk)

Printed in the United States of America

This book is dedicated to all Craig Hospital patients, past, present and future.

Let's Roll!

Contents

List of Illustrations

Acknowledgements

I would like to thank my editor Faye Quam Heimerl for her patience and fortitude in putting up with my sporadic work habits and still being able to stay objective and forthright.

A special thank you is for Jill, Michael and Arlene, my daughter, son-in-law and sister, who always have my best interests at heart but also sometimes think and act as if they are my parents.

My hearty thanks goes to the Craig Hospital staff for allowing me to interrupt their jam-packed schedules in order to acquire much of the factual data contained in this book. In particular I want to thank Dennis O'Malley and Kenny Hosack who, at the start of this book endeavor had their offices temporarily relegated to the basement of the Patient & Family Housing building, but were still always available to assist me in getting information.

To the many staff, patients and families who shared their stories with me I am sincerely grateful. A special thank you for added assistance goes to Ginny Wood, Barbara Ford, Debbie Arellano, Dana Lee, Terry Chase, Barb Page, Jaime Hoffman, Frank Ramirez, Drew and Jeanie Wills, Courtney and Millie Ferrall, Mark and Alissa Gedman, Amanda Vargo, Earl Rodriguez and Dave Denniston.

Most of all I would like to thank Kenny Hosack for his extraordinary assistance in providing access to Craig staff, data and archived information and for his astute suggestions (requested or not) that made writing *No Whining* so much fun and so rewarding.

Preface

"Your chances of walking again are between Poor and Fair, about 40%."

—Dr. Shih-Fong Hsu

I originally intended to write this book from my journals at Craig Hospital where, as a patient on the SCI (Spinal Cord Injury) floor, I kept a log of my progress and recorded my impressions of the staff, facilities, patients and many daily occurrences.

This strategy worked just fine for a previous book I'd written, *Where's The Runway? And Other Flying Stories* (iUniverse, 2001). I simply reviewed my logbooks to refresh my memory and then started writing about incidents—comical and serious—that had occurred during my 30 years of piloting small airplanes and hot air balloons. If I intended to do justice to my description of the unique and inspiring environment epitomized by the "No Whining" sign hanging in the Craig 3West gym—I knew I needed to take a different approach.

Primarily Craig Hospital is an institution of higher learning, a university-level educational center, an academy. Despite its name, Craig Hospital is only a hospital by necessity. At Craig, *rehabilitation* means adaptation through education, an education that starts upon admittance and continues throughout life. All staff members—doctors, nurses, med techs, lab technicians, physical therapists, occupational therapists, housekeepers, and even maintenance workers—are educators. Patients and their families are students. (Upon discharge Craig patients are even called "Graduates" and become members of an active alumni association.)

I can only hope my words manage to convey even a little of the magnitude of what Craig Hospital did for me, with me, and I can also only hope to inspire SCI patients to keep trying, to believe in what can be accomplished through planning, hard work, research, education, social environment, camaraderie, building design, adequate resources and interpersonal interaction.

It is my wish that you will enjoy this book and, more importantly, that you come away with a focused, positive outlook on what the future can be for Craig Hospital and the treatment of SCI.

To provide assistance and direction for those who wish to obtain further information concerning spinal cord injuries, I have included a list of abbreviations and glossary of words and terms used in *No Whining* as well as a bibliography of written materials and websites used in its preparation.

Abbreviations

ACU	Acute Care Unit
BP	Blood Pressure
BWI	Baltimore-Washington International Airport
Cath	A catheter; to catheterize
COTA	Certified Occupational Therapist Assistant
DIA	Denver International Airport
EMT	Emergency Medical Technician
ER	Emergency Room
IC	Intermittent Catheterization; self-catheterization
Meds	Medications
MRI	Magnetic Resonance Imaging
MSPT	Master of Science in Physical Therapy
NIDRR	National Institute on Disability and Rehabilitation Research
OT	Occupational Therapy; Occupational Therapist
PT	Physical Therapy; Physical Therapist
RMRBIS	Rocky Mountain Regional Brain Injury System
RMRSIS	Rocky Mountain Regional Spinal Injury System
RN	Registered Nurse
RPT	Registered Physical Therapist
SCI	Spinal Cord Injury
SOP	Standard Operating Procedure
TBI	Traumatic Brain Injury

TM   Transverse Myelitis

TR   Therapeutic Recreation

1

An Injury Gets Me to Craig

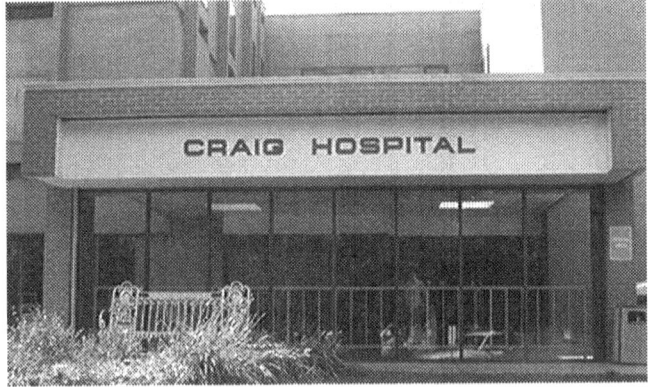

Fig. 1–1

The weekend started out exactly as planned. After leaving my car Friday afternoon at the long-term parking lot at Denver International Airport, I easily passed through security and once I was seated in a Frontier Airbus I fell into a deep sleep. I was headed towards Baltimore-Washington International Airport.

The plane landed ten minutes ahead of schedule but I was in no hurry to pick up my rental car for the half-hour or so drive from the airport to my hotel in Annapolis, Maryland where I planned to meet Olivia, my friend from Florida, and then attend her cousin's wedding on Sunday afternoon. I planned to head back to Colorado on an early Monday morning flight. Thanks to Olivia's invitation bringing me to Maryland, I was eagerly looking forward to having Saturday lunch with Bill Shepard and his wife, Lois. Bill and I had been bunk counselors together at Camp Takajo, a boys' summer camp located in Naples, Maine, and had not seen each other or been in touch since the summer of 1958. Through one of the wonderful benefits of the Internet—and sheer luck—we had been reunited. Camp Takajo, founded in 1947 and still going strong, maintains a website with a guest book and through this website feature we found each other, discovering that, among other coincidences, we were both newly published authors using the same publisher. I was really looking forward to seeing Bill again, meeting Lois and catching up on all those years.

It was a typical December Maryland night, dark and raining and, as I headed toward Annapolis, I wondered whether I would be able to see the road signs and get off at the correct exit or would I end up taking an unwanted tour of the Eastern coast. Luckily I easily navigated the exit. Finding the hotel was not so easy as it is tucked between two buildings on the main street and, due to the rain and my sixty-seven-year-old fading eyesight, I drove right by it. I executed a "missed approach"—a flying term—, circled the block for another try and this time found the hotel's courtyard entrance. After checking in, I entered my room and plopped down on the bed, wiped out.

The next morning I awoke to sunshine and slightly cool temperatures which, I was told, was still quite warm for Maryland in the middle of December. After shaving, showering and dressing, I made my obligatory check-in telephone call to my daughter back in Denver to assure her I was fine, in the right hotel and had not forgotten anything, Then I joined Olivia for a walk to find a place for breakfast.

After a brisk walk ending only a few blocks from the hotel, we found a small coffee shop where we sat down to a light breakfast and I read the local newspaper which I found interesting but, being unfamiliar with local events, was totally unaware of what and who they were reporting about. I left the paper on the table along with, for me, a generous tip and, trying my best to remember where I had parked the rental car the previous evening, and also trying to recall what make, model and color it was, we headed back to the hotel. At Olivia's excellent suggestion, I pushed the button on the car's key chain and, thanks to the beeping horn and flashing lights, I found that the car was exactly where I'd left it.

Bill and Lois lived quite a distance east of Annapolis so we decided to split the distance and meet in between at Grasonville. In the car's glove compartment I found the Mapquest map I had downloaded from the Internet, and, after studying it for a few moments, we drove out of the hotel garage and found our way to Highway 50, and headed east towards Grasonville where Bill and I had arranged to meet for lunch.

We drove with the windows slightly open to enjoy the salt air of Chesapeake Bay and, despite being in unfamiliar territory, actually found the right highway exit and arrived at the Fisherman's Inn and Crab Deck restaurant a little early.

We found seats in the empty waiting area near the entrance to await Bill and Lois' arrival. I hoped I would somehow recognize Bill after 46 years.

We waited about fifteen minutes, nervously eyeing a number of people who came through the door. No one looked familiar. Finally a couple walked in and one look told me they were Bill and Lois. I knew Bill right away. Sure, Bill appeared a little older looking but he was still tall, thin (thinner than me, for sure) and hadn't lost those unforgettable bushy eyebrows. He also had that mischievous twinkle in his eye that I clearly remembered from that summer at Camp Takajo so long ago.

Bill, Lois, Olivia and I ate Maryland crab cakes while Bill and I rehashed old times when we ate lobsters in Maine, recounted stories of our youth and filled each other in on where we had been for the last 46 years. We discussed our budding writing careers, mine consisting of one book on my flying adventures and another one an anthology of five stories each from myself and five other Colorado authors. Bill's consisted of an adventure novel series paralleling his true-life career in the U.S. Foreign Service and a book on wine.

After passing a couple of hours together, we said our goodbyes and left each other with a promise to stay in touch. Olivia and I headed back to Annapolis to relax and socialize with some of the other wedding guests who were staying at the same hotel.

I slept late Sunday morning. There was no rush to get to the wedding anyway, as it was scheduled to start at 12:00 noon and was only a five-minute drive from the hotel. Taking full advantage of the hotel's services, I spoiled myself by ordering a light breakfast from Room Service. After finishing breakfast and trying hard to shake off an attack of laziness, I showered, dressed and went to the lobby to meet Olivia and some guests who had asked to drive to the wedding with us.

I avoided any possible problems finding the car this time by using the valet service. Then, following clear and easy written directions I left the hotel and got us to our destination in only four minutes, forty-five seconds. The directions were only off by 15 seconds. Feeling fine, there was no indication of any problems and I had no reason to even think of any health issues.

The pre-ceremony reception was excellent and I walked around, mingling with the other guests and enjoying the buffet of fruit, scrambled eggs, small toast pieces, and other familiar and some not-so-familiar food offerings. The wedding ceremony was elegant and, afterward, everyone was ushered into a large room where the band was already playing and the tables beautifully set with place cards at the designated, numbered tables. I found my card and, not wanting to sit with my back to the band, switched cards with someone else and sat down to enjoy the meal, dancing and especially to enjoy the festivities surrounding Uri and Sarah's marriage.

Within an hour after being seated, I noticed a strange tingling that started in my right foot and extended to my ankle. It was barely noticeable and I shrugged it off as a reaction to the medication I was taking to treat Parkinson's disease. Diagnosed a few years earlier, my Parkinson's disease was still considered mild and had not given me any problems previously except for some minor hand tremors.

Soon, there was *more than tingling* in my right foot; there was *definite* numbness. I thought my shoes must have been too tight. (Because of where I lived—in the Colorado High Country town of Breckenridge—I only needed one suit and one pair of black leather shoes, both of which I wear only once every couple of years.) I removed my right shoe but the feeling in my foot didn't return. I began to worry.

Okay then, if the numbness wasn't from a pinching shoe, then surely it was Parkinson's related—at least that's what I thought. I got up from the table and walked to the men's room but my balance was not right. Was my medicine doing this? I checked my prescription dosage and it appeared to be in order.

Later, after a light dinner with Olivia I took a short walk. Now not only were my right ankle and foot numb, but my legs were stiff too. Since I was going back to Denver the next morning, I used my cell phone to try to set up an appointment with my neurologist in Denver instead of seeing a doctor in Baltimore, and hoped the answering service did its job.

Once back at my room, I packed my suitcase then climbed up on the bed to watch TV, mellow out and get some sleep, but after two or three hours of alternately watching TV and snoozing, I headed for the bathroom that was across the room. This was when I *knew* I had problems. I couldn't walk without holding on to a piece of furniture.

Still naively thinking my problem was Parkinson's related, I drew a hot bath. I assumed the hot water would improve the blood circulation in my legs and make me able to walk properly again. I thought, *now I'm for sure going to see my Neurologist in the morning*.

After relaxing in the bath for about 15 minutes and getting some relief from the numbness in my legs, I decided to try to get some sleep. I'd worry about everything in the morning. So, after getting out of the bathtub I went over to the toilet to urinate, but I couldn't, as I had no muscular urge to do so. Again, I ignored an obvious sign of trouble and instead stumbled my way back to bed for some much needed sleep.

I'd set my alarm for 4:30am, so I could get ready and return the rental car to Baltimore in time to make my scheduled 7:30am departure to Denver. I slept fitfully and woke up before the alarm went off. I didn't make my flight.

Getting out of bed and planning to go to the bathroom to do what one does the first thing in the morning, I took a step and began to fall. If I hadn't grabbed a chair I would have gone down. Not only was my right foot numb now, but also my right leg, my left foot, my left leg and my pelvic region. I couldn't move my legs or even wiggle my toes. It felt like my lower body was encased in cold cement. No way could I blame this on poor circulation.

I called Olivia and, trying to suppress my rising panic, asked her to call the front desk and tell them there was a medical situation in room 224 that required a wheelchair and immediate transportation to the nearest hospital. A few minutes later someone from the front desk called to say the hotel's bellman would be right up to my room to help me. Still having full mobility and strength in my upper body, I was able to struggle into my pants, socks and shoes and was ready when the bellman arrived with a wheelchair.

The bellman let himself in with his passkey then helped me from the bed into the wheelchair. Although I didn't know it, time was of the essence and I couldn't have been luckier. My bellman happened to be an EMT working a second job at the hotel.

The EMT had his medical bag with him and a clipboard holding a questionnaire to be completed for the emergency room doctors. He checked my vital signs, asked me about my symptoms, any medications I'd taken and about any possible drug allergies I might have then took me downstairs and helped me get into the hotel's Land Rover.

As the EMT drove out of the hotel's parking lot, he told me that one of Maryland's best emergency and trauma hospitals, The Anne Arundel Medical Center, was only three minutes away. He got me there in less than two minutes.

Since I had already been triaged by a hospital EMT—my bellman and driver—I was immediately wheeled into a room and examined by Dr. Young, the attending emergency room physician. He told me that my condition was probably Guillaume-Barre Syndrome and was definitely not Parkinson's related. He assured me he'd already put in a call to the staff neurologist on duty.

Within a half hour Neurologist Jackie Syme MD arrived to examine me. He ordered some blood tests, a lumbar tap and Foley catheterization to empty my now full and paralyzed bladder. After performing some reflex tests and some muscle sensitivity and pressure awareness tests, Dr. Syme confirmed the paralysis. He advised me that it would take a little while to come up with a specific diagnosis, but since I hadn't experienced any physical trauma, the physicians present had already narrowed the possibilities to a few diseases. These possibilities included Rocky Mountain Spotted Fever, Lyme Disease, West Nile Virus, Transverse Myelitis and Guillaume-Barre Syndrome, none of which I knew anything about or liked the sound of.

Despite my growing anxiety, I watched with indifference as the ER techs and nurses painlessly inserted the Foley Catheter and I lay still as Dr. Syme performed a lumbar tap. Fortunately, the hospital has a laboratory on the premises and the spinal fluid from the tap was analyzed within minutes.

While waiting for the lab results, Dr. Syme explained that he was leaning towards a diagnosis of Transverse Myelitis or Guillaume-Barre Syndrome. He advised me that one major difference between these two afflictions was this: If my diagnosis was Transverse Myelitis, it meant the paralysis would probably stop at or near my waist. If, on the other hand my diagnosis was Guillaume-Barre Syndrome, it meant there was a good chance the paralysis could work its way up to my neck, thus paralyzing my lungs. Dr. Syme assured me that if the latter was the case, the Emergency Respiratory Team was standing by ready to intubate me. The only thing the ER staff could do for the next hour or so was closely monitor me for changes.

For the next three hours I lay in a bed in the Anne Arundel Medical Center Emergency Room, fighting panic and dreading the thought of having tubes shoved down my throat. I constantly poked my finger into my stomach, chest, lower back and shoulders to test for sensation and make sure no numbness was occurring.

Every twenty minutes or so, Dr.Syme returned to the ER to stab or scratch me with some kind of small, sharp instrument. If I felt discomfort, the paralysis hadn't spread. Dr. Syme's poking and scratching eventually ended, but not before my torso looked like someone had played a series of Tic-Tac-Toe games all over it.

My stay in the emergency room lengthened to ten hours, during which time my paralysis did not creep any higher than my waist. At this point, Dr. Syme and his fellow ER doctors concluded I'd contracted Transverse Myelitis and ordered an MRI to help verify their diagnosis. I was immediately started on steroids to halt the inflammation of my spinal cord and within minutes I was admitted as a patient to the Anne Arundel Medical Center's Acute Care Unit (ACU).

In the meantime, Olivia had canceled my return flight reservation for Denver as well as her own for Florida and appraised my daughter Jill of my situation. Jill immediately made plans to come to Annapolis the next day.

Once I was settled in at the ACU, the steroid treatment began in earnest but physical therapy was not started, as I was too medically unstable to commence a proper physical therapy plan. Again, I felt no pain, sickness or weakness, only the mental stress associated with realizing that *I was a Paraplegic*. How does a person tell himself he may never walk again? The enormity of my probable massive lifestyle change loomed but I wasn't cognizant of it…yet.

Dr. Syme's prognosis for recovery from TM was gloomy. TM patients' recovery rate ranged from 5% to 100%, dependent upon their age, health and how soon after the SCI occurs does intensive physical therapy start. I struck out on all three conditions as I was in the upper age bracket with Parkinson's disease and could not start physical therapy.

I was determined to prove the doctors wrong, but this was easier said than done, as I knew my stay at Anne Arundel Medical Center was temporary and I would soon be looking for a more permanent rehabilitation hospital. My daughter Jill was way ahead of me. She and Dr. Ian Levenson, my family physician, were already hard at work on the telephone making arrangements for me to transfer to Craig Hospital in Englewood, Colorado.

It just so happens that Craig is one of the premier SCI rehabilitation hospitals in the United States, and it also just so happens to be located only minutes away from Jill's house. Despite the fact that a nationally known TM rehabilitation clinic was located at Johns Hopkins University in nearby Baltimore, I wanted to go back to Colorado. Facing at least a two-month hospital stay, I wanted to be as close to home as possible.

During my seven days in the ACU at Anne Arundel, and even though I was far from home, I was visited by many friends and acquaintances. My friend Olivia had extended her Maryland stay to be with me. My old camp buddy, Bill Shepard came by. Dr. David Krimmins, the new bride's father, came by the hospital every morning to see how I was doing, and, of course, my daughter Jill flew in from Denver and stayed with a friend nearby.

Jill and I had hoped I'd stay a patient at the Anne Arundel Medical Center until my transfer to Craig Hospital came through but my medical insurance company had other plans. I was admitted to Anne Arundel because of a medical emergency and my insurance coverage was only for emergency care. This insurance coverage would terminate when my medical condition had stabilized and I was ready to begin rehabilitation. The most the insurance would pay was for an additional five days.

Despite Herculean efforts by my daughter and Dr. Levenson to get me transferred to Craig Hospital in Denver, they were unsuccessful as there were no open beds at Craig. So Jill and I were forced to make a decision—stay in Maryland and transfer to Johns Hopkins or find another rehab facility in Colorado. My preference was to be close to home so Jill contacted Spalding Hospital in Denver (not too far from Craig Hospital) and the hospital was able to admit me.

My transfer was authorized and shortly thereafter Jill's and my education in "spinal cord injury adaptation" began. Because Jill was flying back to Denver with me, she had the responsibility of checking and draining my catheter bag while we were in the air. A nurse gave her instructions about catheter care as well as other instructions in case any problems arose.

Ready to leave Anne Arundel, I was wheeled into a specially equipped van that could accommodate a wheelchair and, along with my suitcase, left and followed my daughter's car from the hospital to the United Airlines Departure area at Baltimore-Washington International Airport.

The van ride to the airport was painful as my back was sore from sitting in the wheelchair so long. After an extremely uncomfortable ride, we arrived at the United Airlines departure area at BWI and I became very concerned about how I was supposed to get out of the van, through the airport terminal and, most importantly, into my seat on the aircraft. How could I be expected to know these things when only days before I was walking around under my own power?

My concerns were totally without merit because I didn't have to know what to do. The United Airlines personnel had everything under control. They transferred me from the van's wheelchair to the airport's wheelchair and then pushed me to the departure gate and then to the door of the aircraft. United Airlines personnel were not only trained in assisting wheelchair bound passengers, they also had experience in using their training.

After being wheeled to the aircraft door in a standard manual wheelchair, a smaller chair was brought from the aircraft and placed in front of my wheelchair. This smaller chair—an aisle chair—is designed to easily roll down the aisle of the aircraft where a standard size chair would be too wide.

At this point I wondered how I was going to get from my wheelchair into the aisle chair. I weigh over two hundred pounds and could not assist in any way. The only people there were my daughter, two female flight attendants and the United Customer Service Agent. The only people present who weren't trained were my daughter and me. Without hesitation, the flight attendants positioned themselves at my sides, the agent in back and on the count of three they easily lifted me like I weighed nothing and placed me in the aisle chair. With one Flight Attendant in front of the chair and the other in back, they wheeled me smoothly up the aisle to our seats.

Since the flight was not full, United had allowed us to upgrade to First Class to accommodate the situation and make it a little more comfortable for me. The transition from the aisle chair to the wide, First Class seat was smooth and easy for all concerned; especially after they were careful to take proper precautions to protect the catheter leg bag I was wearing from snagging on the seat. Being slightly embarrassed and not having traveled under these conditions before, I was truly surprised at the professionalism and ease with which the airline's personnel worked. Without saying a single word, either to me or to themselves, they accomplished their task quickly.

My daughter told me that she was still trying to arrange for my admission to Craig but needed my records from Maryland and Dr. Levenson's referral. She also told me that she had an appointment in three days to visit Craig Hospital and discuss my situation with the Admissions Department.

After what seemed like an extra long flight from BWI, the plane landed at DIA and again, a well trained team of United Airlines employees easily transferred me from my seat to the aisle chair, from the aisle chair to a wheelchair and finally from the airline's wheelchair to a wheelchair belonging to the handicapped taxi service hired to transport me to Spalding Hospital in Denver.

The ride to Spalding took about thirty minutes and was probably the most uncomfortable ride I have ever had. Sitting strapped in a wheelchair with nothing to hold on to as the van weaved its way through Denver traffic put tremendous pressure on my neck and back muscles causing significant pain and muscle strain. The wheelchair had a very hard seat and evidently was not tied down properly. When we arrived at Spalding I was exhausted, weak and in pain. I'm sure that the admitting nurse thought I was a lot worse off than my chart showed.

Once in my room at Spalding it was fairly easy to settle in to the daily routine, as the staff there is excellent, caring and well trained. They had a number of patients undergoing rehabilitation from various surgeries and there was a group exercise session every afternoon where I met other patients but there were no other spinal cord injury patients.

While I stayed at Spalding (seven days) my daughter Jill was facilitating the completion of all the paperwork necessary to have my case reviewed by the Craig admissions personnel for a decision on whether or not they would accept me as a patient. While waiting for this process to be completed, Jill took the time to drive to Craig Hospital and looked at the facilities. Kenny Hosack, Director of Provider Relations, guided her on this tour of the Craig complex. After the tour, she came to visit me at Spalding and said: "If your case fits the criteria and is accepted for the program at Craig, that's where you're going, Period!"

Three days later Craig Hospital's Dr. Shih-Fong Hsu called me to say that treating TM patients is one of their specialties and that a bed would be available for me within 24 hours. A day and a half later, after another short, painful and exhausting van ride, I arrived at Craig Hospital and began an incredible eight week program that has not only changed my thinking and understanding of SCI and TBI but has, in a very positive way, changed my approach to life in general.

2

Spinal Cord Injury: The Reality

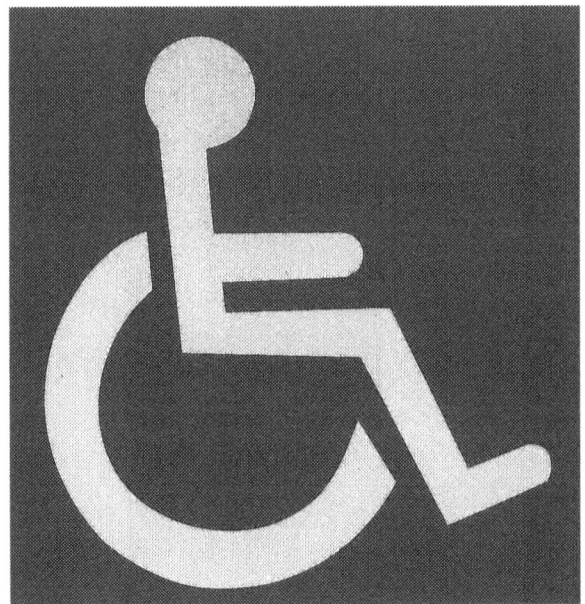

Fig. 2–1

Like most people, I had never given spinal cord injury (SCI) more than an occasional thought and then usually only in response to a news account of an accident or after meeting someone who was in a wheelchair due to an injury. Actor Christopher Reeve's horseback riding accident in 1995 brought SCI to the news forefront but, other than articles I read regarding his treatment, research and possible treatment advances, I really didn't pay much attention to the day-to-day challenges people with spinal cord injuries—and their caregivers—face.

After I transferred from the medical area, 3West, in which I stayed for 4 days, to the rehabilitation area, 3East, the realization that I was no longer an *observer* of people with SCI but someone *with* SCI hit me. This was more than hard to accept at first, but soon, facing the daily challenges of SCI became a regular part of my life.

Shortly after I moved to 3East, Terry Chase, Patient & Family Education Program Coordinator, visited me. She welcomed me to Craig then plopped an enormous three ring binder titled *Spinal Cord Injury Handbook* on my tray and said, "I suggest you start on page one." I gaped at her and she nodded, yes, she was serious. Terry's amazing impact on my rehabilitation is discussed in a later chapter.

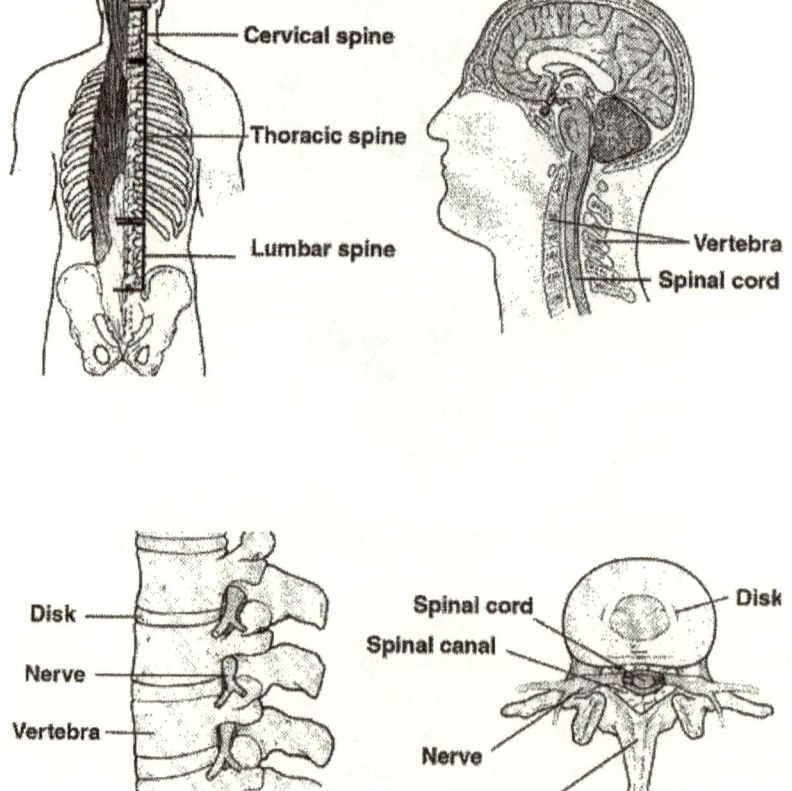

Fig. 2-2

The *Handbook* reminded me of long ago science courses in which I was taught that the spinal cord is an extension of the brain and acts as a conduit from the brain to all parts of the body. The spinal cord transmits two-way messages between the brain and the muscles, internal organs, the skin and other body parts. The spinal cord consists of a bundle of nerve fibers from which nerve cells emanate and when connected to the brain form the two main divisions of the central nervous system.

Messages moving *from* the brain *to* the muscles control movement. Interrupt these messages with SCI and there is paralysis. Messages moving *from* the body *to* the brain provide sensation (or feelings) such as pain, temperature, pressure, etc. Interrupt these messages to the brain and there's loss of sensation.

The extent of bodily function loss from SCI depends on where the spinal cord is injured. The higher up the spinal cord the injury occurs, the greater the loss of function of not only muscles but also organs located below the injury. This can mean loss of bladder, bowel or sex organ function. Paradoxically, the spinal cord may continue to function below the injury but messages to the brain are interrupted and some patients will incur involuntary exaggerated reflex actions that were previously brain controlled.

The spinal cord is located in the spinal canal and is protected by bones called vertebrae that are held together by muscle and other tissue with this total area being known as the spinal column. Nerve cells exit the spinal canal between the vertebrae and below their spinal cord segments. The four segment areas are the cervical (neck), thoracic (chest), lumbar (lower back) and sacral (tailbone) with each area containing a certain number of vertebrae and spinal nerves. In my case, the injury (where the virus lodged) was in the thoracic (T) segment near the 10th vertebrae, resulting in T-10 Paraplegia.

Injuries to the spinal cord usually occur in two ways, physical trauma and illness. Physical trauma, the most common type of SCI, can be a result of an auto accident, diving accident, gunshot wound, sports injury, a fall and the like. SCI caused by illness can come from spinal diseases, the aging process or from an inflammation.

Transverse Myelitis (TM) is a disease in which inflammation of the spinal cord causes the spinal cord to swell and prevent messages from traveling in the spinal cord. It can also damage nerve endings there. Blocked messages combined with damaged nerve endings result in paralysis and loss of sensation. The extent of nerve damage cannot be ascertained until after the inflammation has subsided. The prognosis for recovery also cannot be ascertained—if at all—until the inflammation has subsided. Sometimes damaged nerve cells recover, but if they don't, the patient could have permanent loss of various functions.

Even with the *Spinal Cord Injury Handbook* information right in front of me I still couldn't quite accept my circumstances; I needed to know more. I used the computer Internet facilities available to Craig patients to surf the web and I located several technical TM sites as well as some reader-friendly TM sites. All seemed to agree on a number of points about TM:

1. There's only three or four reported cases of TM per million of the population. (With these odds I would have preferred to win the lottery.)

2. TM's cause is still unknown but statistics point to a viral infection as the prime suspect. The virus itself damages the spinal cord, and so too can the body's immune response to the virus.

3. TM symptoms can appear suddenly and reach their peak very quickly or they can develop slowly over a period of weeks.

4. The recovery rate ranges from ten percent to almost one hundred percent.

5. The time between onset and maximum recovery ranges from six months to three years.

6. TM treatment starts with drug intervention to reduce inflammation and follows with vigorous physical therapy rehabilitation as soon as medically possible.

7. Most studies agreed the rate of recovery and length of time for recovery are directly related to how soon intense physical therapy commences after the injury occurs.

Finding out there *was a chance* for substantial recovery did little to assuage what I felt as I lay in a bed unable to turn my lower body which felt like it was encased in cool cement. My feet seemed to be wearing wool socks inside of tight ski boots. I was terrified.

Being a former hockey player and still active athletically, the realization that I couldn't so much as wiggle my toes or feel anything below my waist was almost too much, but what really rattled my cage, was the thought of giving up my home.

I live in a three-story town house where traversing the three staircases and getting around the house in a wheelchair is impossible. Where would I live upon discharge if I couldn't go home? The only feasible option at the moment was to live with my daughter near Craig Hospital; however, the thought of trying to maneuver around her house with my two small grandsons chasing me gave me heartburn.

As I lay in my hospital bed on Craig Hospital's floor 3West I just couldn't get comfortable. I wasn't sick or in pain, just stressed and completely exhausted from my ordeal in Annapolis and the moves from Anne Arundel Medical Center to Spalding Hospital and finally to Craig Hospital.

Adding to my stress were side effects from the medications I was now taking, probably the steroids. First off, my vision changed, enough so that I needed new reading glasses and for the first time I needed glasses for distance vision. Dr. Hsu advised me to wait to get new glasses until I was weaned off the steroids, as my vision would probably correct itself then.

The second side effect of the steroids was scary—at first. If I stared at an object for a few seconds the object grew legs and wiggled around like a psychedelic millipede in brilliant color. The first time this happened I was lying in bed while still at Spalding Hospital and staring at the pipes under the sink in my room. At first, I thought there was a large insect on the pipes but soon realized I was hallucinating. I then stared at the light switch on the far wall and the same thing happened. My fear turned to pleasure. After that, whenever I was bored, I just stared at a ceiling tile or door handle and watched it grow legs and wiggle. (Sure enough, after I was weaned off the steroids, my wiggly hallucinations disappeared.)

As if paralysis, exhaustion and hallucinations weren't enough to push me to wallow in self-pity, knowing I had to accept that I was a paraplegic so that I could begin to recover made me want to "go under" altogether. To accept my condition and thereby fully appreciate the rehabilitation process, would mean I had to lose all shyness, physical inhibition and expectation of privacy. How could I give up the privacy that I'd grown accustomed to over a lifetime of self-sufficiency and fierce independence.

I had been hospitalized before and was familiar with the miserable conditions of depending on a catheter to assist my bladder functions; and on oxygen and mechanical assistance for breathing. Of course that was uncomfortable, but worst than that (for me, anyway), was the embarrassment of having to use a bed pan for bowel movements.

The inability to take care of myself made me angry, yet knowing I was in a hospital environment seemed to calm me. But then again, being dependent on Craig techs to empty my catheter bag, wipe my rear, turn me in bed, wash me and provide almost every other basic need, brought on an almost indescribable sadness. How could I possibly perform basic functions for myself? How could I dress, eat or go to the mall, much less drive a car or play golf. What if I became a burden on my family? How could I have a future now? I couldn't comprehend. My concerns were sapping both my mental and physical strength.

After a day of being left alone to sleep and recover some strength, I rode in a wheelchair to the 3West gym. There I met a physical therapist and an occupational therapist and underwent a series of tests to determine my physical strength, agility, balance and specifically what functions and sensations had been lost. The results of these tests were then made a part of my records and formed the basis for a complete diagnosis and prognosis.

Ten days after I was admitted to Craig I was invited to a conference for the purpose of officially discussing my test results and putting my medical diagnosis and my prognosis for recovery on the record. The conference became the turning point of my Craig experience.

The following people attended the conference: my daughter Jill and her husband Michael, my sister Arlene (by telephone), Dr. Shih-Fong Hsu MD (Rehab Team Leader), Jaime Hoffman (caseworker), Donna Rainford (occupational therapist), Hugh Simson (physical therapist), Debbie Shultz (nurse) and psychologist Toby Huston.

Dr. Hsu chaired the conference and each department representative discussed the type of tests performed and the results and prognosis. Except for the neutral or positive reports from nursing, my caseworker and the psychologist, all reports were slightly negative. Evidently, I had less upper body strength and poorer muscle reflex action in my legs than I thought.

Dr. Hsu spoke last, describing TM and discussing the intense physical rehabilitation I'd need to undergo and the hard work I'd have to put in to recover. He stated that the prognosis terms were "Good, Fair and Poor." His diagnosis put me in the lower "Fair" or upper "Poor" range, meaning my chances for a full recovery were poor. I probably would never walk or regain control of my lost functions.

I desperately tried to hold back my tears and not make a complete fool of myself but I was unsuccessful. The silence that ensued seemed endless. Finally Jill tearfully asked, "Is this prognosis irreversible?" Dr. Hsu assured my daughter and me that the prognosis was based on currently available data and that it would be reviewed almost daily. If there was improvement as I progressed through rehabilitation, my prognosis would be adjusted accordingly.

He said my chances for a full recovery are poor, but he's wrong, I thought, and suddenly a change came over me. I was not going to become a member of the statistical majority. *I'm going to prove him wrong.* I became angry and decided to fight the TM with all my strength.

Ending the conference, Dr. Hsu asked, "Herb, what's your goal for your stay at Craig." I think he expected me to say something about *adapting* to my new environment, but I didn't. He looked very surprised when I announced; "Dr. Hsu, when my discharge day comes, I am going to walk out the door…by myself!"

3

The Craig Philosophy: Experience, Flexibility, & Teamwork

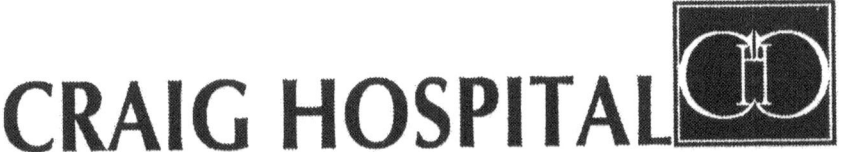

CRAIG HOSPITAL
Caring exclusively for patients with spinal cord and brain injuries.

Fig. 3–1

Within days of my arrival at Craig, my room became as busy as Grand Central Station during rush hour! As one might imagine, I became overwhelmed and confused trying to remember who everyone was.

Their daily visits started while I was temporarily assigned to a semi-private room on floor 3West, the older spinal cord injury (SCI) floor and continued after my move to a suite on 3East, the newer SCI area. As it turned out, their visits were designed to give me the opportunity to meet most of my rehabilitation team, and to give my team the opportunity to meet me. My visitors at one time or another were:

- Jaime Hoffman—Patient and Family Service Counselor
- Hugh Simson—Physical Therapist
- Donna Rainford—Occupational Therapist
- Dana Lee—Certified Occupational Therapist Assistant

- Terry Chase—Education Coordinator
- Toby Huston—Psychologist
- Joe Gomez—Director, Therapeutic Recreation
- Sue Phillips—Driving Rehabilitation Specialist
- Karen Mathias—Admissions
- The hospital's Chaplain
- Dr. Hsu
- Day and night shift nurses
- Day and night shift techs

Because teamwork is the core of the Craig philosophy, all patients are assigned their own specific team and team leaders to provide them with the highest level of service. Team leaders are the patients' assigned physicians—usually physiatrists (physicians specializing in rehabilitation medicine)—and the other team members are specialists in other disciplines that include rehabilitation nursing, patient and family services, physical therapy, occupational therapy, and psychology.

When the team members and other staff first visited me, they delivered a mini-lecture about their department's function and what he/she planned to do for me (and in some cases, to me). They also left pamphlets and books for me to study; they assumed, of course, that I had already finished studying the voluminous *Spinal Cord Injury Handbook* previously given me. Out of all the reading materials four books or pamphlets had an immediate and profound effect on my attitude and thoughts about Craig Hospital and ultimately on my rehabilitation. They were: *Patient and Family Orientation Handbook, New Patient Handbook*, the latest issue of Craig's Alumni Magazine, *Movin' On*, and *Pathways to Health: You do have a Choice*.

Reading these four publications as well as spending time absorbing all the information on Craig's website, brought me to the realization that Craig was not the usual hospital I had anticipated finding and that the positive attitudes I had encountered, including both staff and patients, were not random but a result of implementing a carefully planned program based on a well developed working philosophy.

The development of this philosophy, based on long-term experience and the ability to be flexible in many areas, had its beginnings close to 100 years ago in 1907 when Frank Craig started the "Tent Colony of Brotherly Love" in the city of Lakewood, near Denver. This tent city, now the site of a nursing home, was founded to care for indigent men with tuberculosis, a disease prevalent in those days. Many of today's major hospitals and treatment centers in the west, like Craig or The City of Hope in Duarte, California, started as tuberculosis tent cities. The West was popular because Tuberculosis sufferers from the cold, damp climate of the eastern United States seemed to find better relief when they moved to the drier, warmer climate of some western states.

Frank Craig ran the "Tent Colony of Brotherly Love" for seven years until he died of tuberculosis in 1914. The name of the tent colony he founded (now having a number of buildings replacing the tents) changed its name to "Craig Colony." Later, when the occurrence of tuberculosis had declined because of recent widespread use of antibiotics, Craig's emphasis turned to treating victims of Muscular Dystrophy, Polio, Multiple Sclerosis and Spinal Cord Injuries.

In 1957, Dr. John Young, MD became Craig's Medical Director and solidified Craig's move to become a center for spinal cord injury and brain injury rehabilitation. "Craig Colony" was then renamed "Craig Rehabilitation Center" to reflect the change in mission. Still later, its name was changed again, this time to "Craig Rehabilitation Hospital." Dr. Young's leadership and treatment philosophies were carried forward and are considered largely responsible for Craig's success today.

Having made the decision to specialize in spinal cord injury (SCI) and traumatic brain injury (TBI) rehabilitation, Craig formed an alliance with Swedish Hospital. In 1970, Craig completed an 80-bed rehabilitation hospital on the grounds of Swedish Hospital, located in the city of Englewood at Hampden Avenue and Clarkson Street. In order to allow Craig patients access to radiology, laboratory, surgery and other medical services at Swedish, Craig and Swedish were connected to each other by a tunnel.

Three years later Craig modified the apartments located across the street from the facility for use as transitional living housing for patients (many patients are ready to leave the hospital environment but are not ready to live independently in their homes.) and for use as housing for inpatients' families. This modification furthered Craig's philosophy of total involvement in rehabilitation.

In 1975, Craig's Board of Directors renamed the facility "Craig Hospital" to reflect the totality of medical and rehabilitation services it now provided. This name remains today.

In 1983, Craig advanced its philosophy of total involvement once again and completed a 62,000 square foot expansion to what is now the West Building.

This expansion included an outpatient clinic, media studio, therapy areas, department offices, and a large gymnasium.

In 1996, Craig brought its treatment philosophy even closer to full potential when it completed construction of what is now the East Building which was designed to maximize contact between patients and staff and between patients and patients. This building houses innovative single-person suites for "transitional" patients, multiple treatment areas, a TBI gymnasium, and research and business office space. It also has a two-level skybridge spanning Clarkson Street connecting the East Building with the West Building.

As recently as 2002, Craig replaced the aging apartments with a new, state of the art, 47-unit Outpatient and Family Housing Facility. This facility houses re-evaluation and transitional patients as well as families of inpatients.

Craig's patient statistics clearly indicate Craig's successful meld of its philosophy of "total involvement in rehabilitation" with its physical structure and infrastructure. Craig averages 425 inpatient admissions, including patients from all 50 states and numerous foreign countries and sees 1600 outpatients every year. All told, Craig has served 25,000 patients since 1956.

Craig's successful meld of philosophy with physical structure and infrastructure is also indicated by its licenses, accreditations, designations and ratings. Craig is:

- Licensed by the State of Colorado as an Acute Care Hospital

- Accredited by the Joint Commission on Accreditation of Healthcare Organizations (JCAHO)

- Designated as a Model System Center (both for SCI and TBI) by the National Institute on Disability and Rehabilitation Research (NIDRR)

- A recipient of Magnet Recognition by the American Nurses Credentialing Center—only the second rehabilitation hospital in the United States to receive this recognition

- One of the top ten rehabilitation hospitals in the United States for 16 consecutive years as rated by US News and World Report

- The first hospital in North America chosen for the FDA Phase II Activated Macrophage Clinical Trial

- Noted for its 49 years of free-standing specialized SCI and TBI rehabilitation and research

As I stated, the physical layout of the SCI floors 3East (Fig. 3–3) and 3West as well as the physical layout of the entire Craig campus (Fig. 3–2) play a vital role in implementing the Craig rehabilitation philosophy. I know this layout had a major impact on my responses to the challenges I faced at Craig.

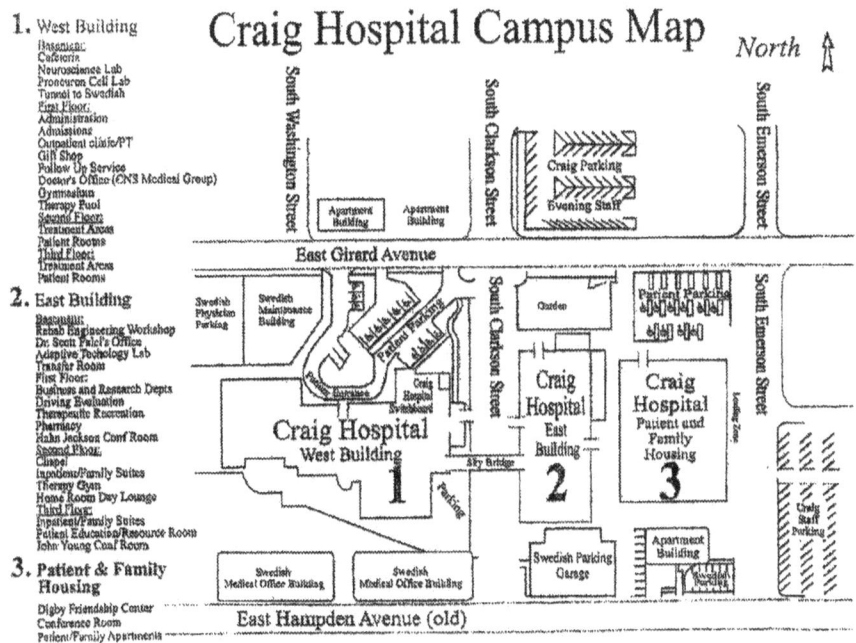

Fig. 3–2

3West, the older floor I was temporarily assigned to, was designed like your typical semi-private hospital room of the 1970s, painted pale blue and with provisions for two patients per room and two rooms per bathroom. (It was anticipated that most patients would not need the use of the bathroom as they were totally immobile anyway).

The individual patient rooms on 3West, painted a light blue with darker blue trim, open onto hallways—mazes, really—lit with fluorescent lighting. The halls all inevitably lead to the nurses' station, elevators, and the therapy gym. Whenever I explored this maze in my wheelchair, I always seemed to get myself lost among a slew of offices, conference rooms and storage areas on the far side of

3West. Once I homed in on the hum of the elevators, I was saved, and I could find my way back to my room.

The patient rooms and total physical layout of 3East, on the other hand, are the exact opposite of 3West. Painted a brighter shade of white, all patient rooms are actually suites with a bedroom area, bathroom, and a large, carpeted room containing a table, three arm chairs, one easy chair, a sofa bed, a sink, a microwave and a refrigerator. All patient rooms on 3East are constructed on outside walls that give each patient a full outside view through an entire wall of windows. Each room has a private bathroom that includes a toilet, a sink and a shower large enough to easily accommodate a wheelchair. The rooms on either end of each floor open into a well-lit hallway and the rooms in the center of the floor open into a large common area furnished with sofas, chairs and a large table. This common area, also called the party room, is used by patients, staff and visitors, and is the site for various social functions such as discharge parties and birthday parties, etc.

The 3East Nurses' Station, at the south end of the common area, is a large, open area with a front counter behind which there is a work area and a limited access pharmacy room where each shift's staff prepares and stores medications required for their shift, eliminating the need for frequent calls and trips to the hospital pharmacy which, of course, is never located near the patients.

The design of 3East is intended to maximize Craig's philosophy that socialization helps eliminate feelings of isolation. Every person, whether going to the elevators at the north end of the floor, the skybridge on the south end, the nurses' station in the center or the education/TV/computer room on the west wall, will pass every other person going in the opposite direction. If you were on your way to a regularly scheduled appointment and others were doing likewise, you would pass the same people at the same time every day. Craig staff members always seem to say "Hello" and "You look great today," (even if you don't) so their greetings become infectious. Soon, I found myself greeting and often talking to staff, other patients and even visitors whom I didn't even know.

Craig's visitation policy, unlike any hospital visitation policy I had ever experienced, also reflects its philosophy of flexibility. Simply put, there are no visiting hours at Craig Hospital. (That's unusual, I know) Visitors may come any time they choose as long as it's not late at night and as long as their visit doesn't interfere with the other patients' sleep.

The policy has one caveat, however—their visit will not, under any circumstance, disrupt or impede the patient's rehabilitation schedule in any way. Visitors are invited to accompany the patient to whatever class is taking place—wheelchair class, pool therapy, education classes, cooking instruction, recreation, etc. My daughter liked to visit when I was scheduled for Physical Therapy in the gym so she could watch my progress as I learned to walk again. Friends asked for my pool therapy schedule so they could get a laugh from my attempts to balance myself on an underwater beam in neck deep water. They always refused the invitation to join me in the pool.

Craig's present-day treatment philosophy of flexibility and the ability to adapt quickly to changes, started in 1957 with its decision to specialize in SCI and TBI, has been proven to produce positive outcomes not only for patients, but also for Craig Hospital.

Craig's team approach to treatment, along with its deliberately casual yet professional atmosphere, has resulted in outstanding staff loyalty. Of the approximately 450 full-time and 200 part-time and per-diem staff:

- One third have been at Craig for ten or more years;
- The President, Dennis O'Malley has been at Craig for 33 years;
- The VP of Finance, Ron Branish has been at Craig for 18 years;
- The Medical Director, Dr. Daniel Lammertse, MD has been at Craig for 24 years;
- The Senior VP of Operations, Scott Manley, EdD has been at Craig for 35 years;
- My physician and Team Leader Shih-Fong Hsu, MD has been at Craig for 27 years.

Bolstered by Craig's good employee benefits, recognition programs, seminars, discussion groups and department retreats, every employee strives to maintain a positive and congenial attitude, especially when they are in contact with patients. The fact that the staff feeds off of this positive attitude is readily apparent and this causes the patients to adopt the same attitude.

I am certain Craig's congenial and positive atmosphere was a major reason why what could have been an exercise in gloom and depression while I was a patient there, was instead an experience of hope and accomplishment.

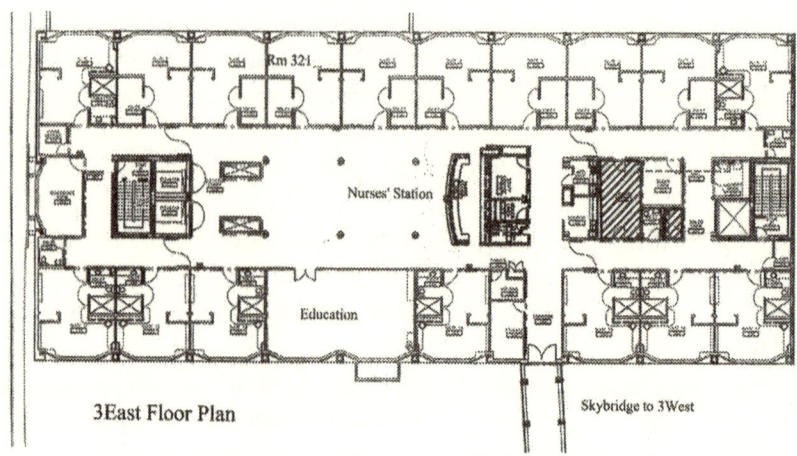

Rm 321

Nurses' Station

Education

3East Floor Plan

Skybridge to 3West

Fig. 3–3

4

Movin' to the East Side

Making Tracks on the East Side!

Your suite on the East side will be ready
for you on ﹦﹦﹦﹦﹦
Your new room number will be 32.1
Please check with your nurse to find out
the time of your move.

It has been our pleasure to care for you,
and we wish you continued progress and
much happiness.

Your 3 West Care Team

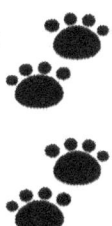

Fig. 4–1

Before arriving at Craig Hospital on December 27, I had already spent four-teen days in two different hospitals; needless to say I was tired and stressed. I was an all-around unhappy camper and eager to check into the deluxe accommodations Jill had described to me the day before. I wanted to get on with things but my room turned out to be the usual humdrum hospital room and a big letdown.

I was wheeled into my semi-private room (the other bed was vacant). I couldn't decide what color the walls were painted since the room was poorly lit, but I narrowed it down to either light gray or light blue. I was certain though, that the moldings were trimmed in dark blue. The bathroom had to be shared with a possible future roommate and also with the two occupants of the next room.

My room was furnished with the standard adjustable hospital bed. It had three position choices but I learned soon enough that none of those choices included any semblance of comfort. Above the bed was a motorized contraption bolted into the ceiling. It had a black t-bar and canvas straps hanging from it, and it seemed to move on rails.

There were also the expected tubes, gauges and mysterious multi-colored pipes sticking out of the wall at the head of the bed. Interestingly there weren't any vital sign monitors to check my blood pressure, pulse and heart rate, at least not that I could see.

I tried out my bed but hadn't even begun to relax when a nurse entered the room pushing a Blood Pressure machine. (This explained the missing monitors). She wrapped the pressure cuff around my upper arm then pushed the start button. The cuff squeezed against my arm and the first of at least two hundred vital sign checks I'd receive during my stay at Craig was over. Next, she took my pulse and slid some weird looking gadget in my ear, noted my temperature and then announced it was time to take my medication.

Swallowing pills three times a day never was my favorite activity, but washing down the seven or eight pills three times a day with Englewood, Colorado's undrinkable city water was torture. It took me a day or two to find out that the only potable water (I exaggerate) came out of drinking fountains or sealed water bottles.

Medication time also included getting injections. Before this bout with TM, injections never used to bother me but then I'd never been given Heparin injections. Heparin is prescribed to prevent blood clots from forming in bedridden patients' legs. Because these patients cannot stand up to aid their circulation, there's a chance clots can form.

To get the best results, Heparin must be injected into the belly. In my case, this really shouldn't have mattered as I was paralyzed from the waist down and didn't feel any pain. What bothered me though, was what my gut looked like. What started out as a series of purple dots on my belly ended up looking like I was wearing a purple cummerbund around my mid-section!

Injections were unpleasant and so was the thought of the upcoming evening's "lifting procedure" associated with getting me to the bathroom for my mandatory bowel program. At Spalding Hospital, the lifting procedure entailed one or two techs physically lifting me from my bed to a wheeled commode. Normally, this wasn't a problem—when strong techs helped me. I had good upper body strength and enough mobility to sit up and push my legs over the side of the bed. Once there, a tech placed a wide canvas belt around my chest to assist in lifting me. One tech would stand in front of me and grab the belt while another tech would stand behind me, grab me under my armpits, and, in one fluid motion they would lift me, pivot, and place me on the "target" chair. (Once, two small techs tried to move me and failed. I sank to my knees then planted my face in the bathroom floor.)

I'd been dreading this procedure all day and at 7:00 p.m. the time of reckoning arrived. My Craig Hospital tech Howard Gonzalez strolled into my room announcing, "Hello Mr. Tabak, ready to use the bathroom?"

Great. I've been looking forward to this all day. "If I have to," I answered.

"What're you wearing that thing for? Going someplace?" Howard pointed at the chest belt I'd put on in anticipation of his visit.

"I *thought* I was going to the bathroom."

"You are," Howard said, "but don't expect me to move you by myself." Howard reached for the "contraption" suspended over my bed and slid it into position right above me.

"What's this?" I asked.

"A Guldmann Lift, basically an electric winch. You'll see a lot of action in this while you're here." Howard unhooked what looked like a canvas jacket from a hook on the back of the outside door. He placed it on my back and looped the front pieces under both thighs, then around to the front and then hooked them to the lift.

Howard pushed a button on the hand control and with a gentle hum of the motor I was lifted up off the bed, swung over to the commode and gently lowered to the seat. I felt like the rescued whale in the movie, "Free Willy." (No wonder my fellow patient Dave Denniston called it the "Free Willy" procedure.)

Wow, what a relief! No more cracking ribs from being lifted under the arms, and, no more unplanned inspections of bathroom floors. I later learned every bed in Craig has a Guldmann Lift above it. This way almost any nurse or tech can safely and efficiently move patients. The lifts not only increase patient comfort, but they also help prevent back injuries in Craig staff.

What's next? I wondered. The answer? The "slide board."

My assigned Physical Therapist (PT) Hugh Simson (MSPT) arrived in my room later that day to introduce himself and to take my measurements for the manual wheelchair I would need. Once finished measuring, Hugh handed me a "slide board," (Fig.4–2) a flat piece of wood that's smooth on one side and has rubber strips (like shower mats) glued on the other.

"You'll need this for wheelchair transfers," he said. It was supposed to help me ease myself from my bed into the wheelchair—"ease" being the operative word.

Hugh demonstrated how to use the slide board to get from my bed into the wheelchair. Easier said than done.

1. Position the wheelchair at a slight right angle to and touching the bed.

2. Lock both sets of wheelchair wheels.

3. Slip one end of the board between the bed and your thighs close to your bottom.

4. Place the other end of the board on the wheelchair seat.

5. Using your arms and upper body, slide down the board and into the wheelchair.

This was simple in theory but difficult in execution. Hugh didn't tell me what *should* have been rule number one: Skin and slide boards do not mix.

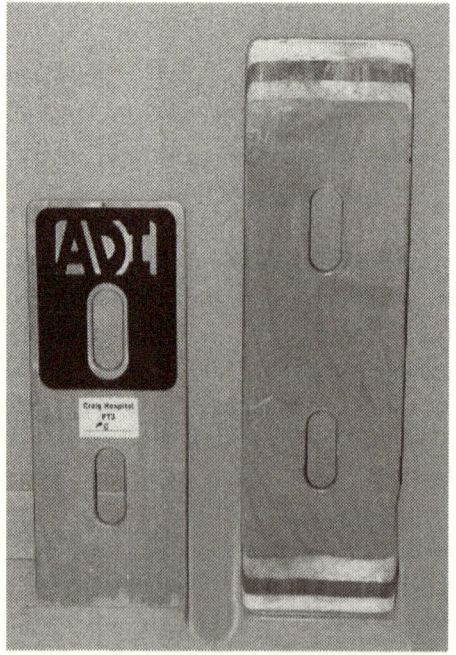

Slide Boards   Fig. 4–2

After a few practice runs, along with a newly raw bottom, I had the technique down good enough for Hugh to "sign me off" wheelchair transfers. There was one condition—a tech had to be standing by to help me if I needed it.

This was great! I had wheels! I could get out of my room and explore the hallway and nearby nurses' station.

Within two days I started to get into the daily routine at Craig. I was still fairly weak, though and the doctors had not yet decided how or if my Parkinson's was going to interfere with my scheduled rehabilitation. I was considered "unstable" so they would not allow me to start the intensive physical therapy that is the crux of Craig's SCI rehab program. I can't say I minded much. I actually enjoyed the lack of stress associated with not being expected to do anything—including talk. I basked in being served my meals in my room and having time to myself. This solitude didn't last very long.

The next morning my tech came in to pick up my breakfast tray and nonchalantly said, "I see you're getting a roommate today."

"Are you sure?" I asked, "I thought there were other vacant rooms. Why can't he go into one of those?"

"The doctors think it would be best for him to be with someone. You're the only one here without a roommate."

Word was he was flying to Denver from somewhere in the South and would arrive later that day. Great!

Sure enough, early that afternoon my new roommate Earl Rodriguez arrived on a gurney pushed by the Air Ambulance flight crew. He'd flown up from Louisiana with his wife and one of his six daughters. I had no idea what his injury was or what kind of shape he was in. I could see his face was very pale and he didn't look too good. He was either sleeping or unconscious so I didn't try to greet him.

When Earl woke up a couple of hours later, I wheeled myself over to his side of the room and introduced myself. He had endured a painful airplane ride so he was tired and sore but had the strength to talk to me. He said his SCI was the result of a gunshot wound and, like me, was paralyzed from the waist down. (*See Earl's story in Chapter 14*).

Earl spent the rest of the day and evening sleeping and I spent my time in my wheelchair building up my strength while I explored 3West. I found elevators, a slew of offices, the visitors' lounge and the gym. I considered my first run successful.

Wheeling my way back to my room I had a near collision with my team Occupational Therapist (OT) Donna Rainford. It was good timing because she needed me to undergo a series of baseline strength tests in the gym. The test results would form the basis for later strength comparisons.

Returning to my room late that afternoon, I found a printed form-note on my bed. The note's heading read, "Making Tracks on the East Side!" It was my moving notice. I was going to 3East. A minute or two later, my daughter Jill walked in and I handed her the note. She read it and then left the room without saying a word. When she returned she was smiling. She'd checked out my new room. "You're going to love the change," Jill said, "but I'll let you decide that for yourself."

I would have vacated my current room in seconds had my nurse not said my move wasn't scheduled until the next day. In the morning, I'd find out what time. Earl was friendly enough, and a good roommate but I wanted my own room. I was excited and relaxed at the same time and I slept better that night than I had in weeks.

The next morning I was up early, scrambling to gather whatever personal items I could reach from my bed. My nurse came in to give me my meds and check my vital signs. My heart rate must have been up because she told me to relax, as it would take a few hours to clean my new room. Its former occupant had just been discharged from Craig that morning. *I don't care if the room's clean, I want to move NOW!* (Of course, I really cared) *"Thanks,"* was all I could think to say.

The hours dragged, I stuck around my room, had lunch in bed, then waited another three hours until about 3 o'clock, I met the man of the hour, Frank Ramirez.

Frank is Housekeeping Supervisor at Craig. He'd come to my room to assure me that the nurse was telling me the truth; my room was being cleaned, but his staff was going to need the rest of the day to finish up.

I couldn't imagine why Housekeeping needed so much time. I was surprised and satisfied to find out that Craig's post patient discharge room cleaning couldn't possibly be any more thorough. Frank explained that the cabinets and shelves (including those in the bathroom) are emptied and everything that's not part of the furniture is taken out of the room.

The bed and mattress are removed, cleaned, sanitized and stored. The room is then disinfected, cleaned and the bedroom area floor is stripped of wax, re-waxed and buffed. The living room/kitchen area carpeting is vacuumed and cleaned. Even the furniture is cleaned. Impressive!

Frank explained that the cleaning would take most of the day but I could plan to move shortly after supper.

Sure enough, just as I was enjoying some watermelon chunks for dessert, my evening tech Howard came in and said, "Let's go for a ride."

He piled all my clothing and other personal items on the bed then disconnected the bed from the electric outlets. As he steered me and the bed toward the door, I called "Goodbye" to Earl. Before Earl could answer, I was whisked from my room and wheeled down the hall and over the glass-enclosed skybridge spanning Clarkson Street. My destination was 3East, Suite 321.

Howard parked my bed under the Guldmann Lift in Suite 321 and left me in the competent care of tech Debbie Arellano and nurse Lilia Smith. Debbie helped me get from my bed into my wheelchair and then gave me a tour of the suite that consisted of three distinct areas:

- A tiled bedroom containing a hospital bed, a moveable night table with drawers, shelves behind the bed, shelves in the wall that divided the bedroom area from the living room area, a wall unit that held a remote controlled TV and VCR and a telephone (with answering machine) on the night table;

- A carpeted living room/kitchen with a wall of larger windows overlooking the Patient and Family Housing and a small parking lot where Adaptive Driving Education vehicles were parked. The area contained a table with three chairs, a lounge chair, a sleeper/sofa, numerous shelves and cabinets, a sink, microwave, refrigerator, and best of all, a high speed computer internet connection;

- A bathroom containing a vanity sink area large enough to store all my toiletries and a generous supply of towels, a commode situated so that a portable commode chair could be placed above it and an open shower area large enough to accommodate a wheelchair, a commode seat or a shower bench.

The suite opened into the visitor/employee/patient lounge area and was directly across from the education Training Room. The Training Room holds two computers available to all patients for Internet use.

Ahh, this was more like the Craig I had heard about. I sighed and with it weeks of stress seemed to ease out of me. Jill was right. I was going to love the changes.

By the time Debbie finished briefing me on my room and giving me a tour of 3East, it was past 9:00pm and Nurse Lilia arrived with my evening meds—and a suggestion.

"I know you're excited about being on 3East," she said, "but I want you to stay calm and get a good night's sleep."

I threw her my best "you've got to be kidding" look. She smiled, "I mean it. Starting tomorrow morning, you're going to be very busy. Rest while you can."

Lilia handed me a copy of my rehab schedule for the remainder of the week and told me that my schedule for each following week would be taped to my door every Friday afternoon. My first days of rehab started at full speed and showed:

- Occupational Therapy sessions starting at 8:00am every day;
- Physical Therapy sessions following each Occupational Therapy session;
- Patient Education group classes every afternoon; and
- Pool Therapy following the Education classes.

I realized I'd be kept busy from 8:00am to 4:00pm, with an hour off for lunch. And I thought I was getting a break from work? Was I ever wrong! Even so, I was glad to be finally able to start therapy. But I was also apprehensive. I didn't know what to expect.

—I wondered if I'd be up for what would be asked of me.

I took in "my" suite one more time, clicked off the light, and effortlessly slipped into a deep sleep. It felt good to be on the East Side.

5

Physical Therapy: Pain & Progress

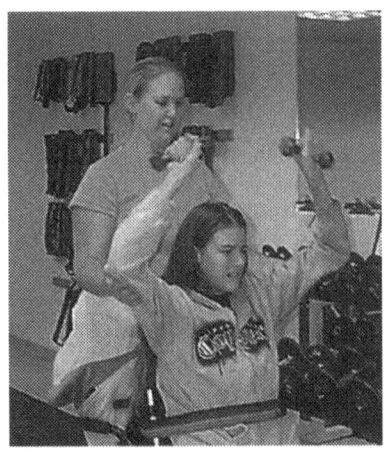

Fig. 5–1

If the team concept is the core of the Craig philosophy then physical therapy is the core of the team concept. When you're lying in bed or sitting in a wheelchair the muscles you don't use rapidly lose elasticity and strength. The goal in SCI rehabilitation is to regain as much muscle use as possible, because if they aren't viable, no amount of nerve recovery can override lost muscle and then recovery becomes extremely difficult. Craig Hospital's physical therapists' primary concern is maximizing patients' muscle viability through strength and mobility therapy. This therapy concentrates on:

- Muscle exercises
- Range of motion exercises

- Aquatic exercises

- Stretching

- Balance and standing

- Slide board transfer instruction and practice

- Mobility and wheelchair skills

My introduction to both Physical and Occupational Therapy at Craig Hospital occurred almost simultaneously and without any wait.

After spending the New Year's holiday weekend resting, exploring every nook and cranny of 3East, visiting with Jill and Michael and playing wheelchair tag with my Grandsons Sam and Zach, I was anxious to start my rehab program. I sure didn't have to wait very long. Although I was anticipating an orientation session with a Physical Therapist, exactly at 8 o'clock Monday morning, Occupational Therapist Joan McMullen knocked on my door and surprised me by starting me on a program that didn't lose its intensity for sixty days.

Joan applied Craig's philosophy of using functional and practical approaches to teaching patients the skills needed to perform independently in the real world. She introduced me to a device known as a "Reacher" (Fig. 5–2)—a handy device to have around even if you're not a paraplegic. It's a long metal rod with a squeeze handle on one end and two grasping "fingers" on the other. It's great for pulling books off of high shelves, retrieving things from the floor and helping you dress yourself. Joan said learning to dress myself was the first order of business. I worked on it for the next four days.

It had been three weeks since I'd been stricken with TM and I still had no feeling or muscle control below my waist. I could barely twitch my toes and it required all my strength and concentration just to raise my right leg about two inches above the mattress. How was I going to put on clothes in this condition?

Joan told me to ignore this "slight problem." The premise was I would never be able to move my lower body and that my only hope for independence was to learn how to dress myself. This seemed like an impossible task but Joan cajoled me into trying. "Have patience. You'll get it."

I adjusted the hospital bed so that I was in a sitting position and watched as Joan demonstrated how to use the reacher to pull up pants and socks. She gave me the go ahead to start dressing which meant putting on my shirt, pants, socks and shoes. (Thank heavens I was wearing underwear.)

I was determined to accomplish this task but didn't have a clue how draining it was going to be. So I snatched some freshly laundered socks and aimed them at my toes.

But what a surprise! Not only couldn't I reach my feet to pull the sock on, I couldn't flex my hips to try to draw my feet closer to my hands. *So that's what the reacher's for,* I thought.

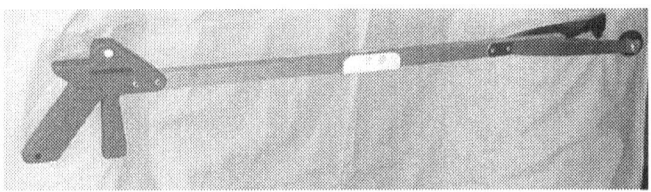

Reacher   Fig. 5–2

By holding the sock in the reacher's fingers, I was able to maneuver my upper body closer to my feet and, stretching as far as I could, swing the sock over my toes and pull it all the way over my foot. Victory!

Yes, victory, but at what price? The entire process of putting on one sock had taken me fifteen minutes and left me exhausted and gulping for air. The second sock went on in faster time—only twelve minutes.

I rested a few minutes then tried using the reacher to pull on my sweat pants. I was a failure from the get-go; I just couldn't coordinate pushing (my legs) and pulling (with the reacher) at the same time. Of course, wearing a leg bag to drain the Foley Catheter didn't help either. What if I pulled the tube out and emptied the bag all over the bed and myself.

The Foley tube stays in the bladder full time but the type of bag it drains into can be changed to fit the circumstances. When a patient is lying in a hospital bed, the tube is constantly draining into a large plastic bag hung on the bed frame. There's a plastic valve located at the bottom of the bag that the techs open in order to drain the urine into a plastic beaker and then dump it into the toilet.

When a patient is ready to actively participate in physical therapy, occupational therapy or education classes, the Foley tube is detached from the bed bag and inserted into a much smaller leg bag which is then strapped to the patient's calf. Because of its smaller size, the leg bag fills much more rapidly than the larger bed bag so it becomes the patient's responsibility to monitor it and inform the tech, nurse or therapist when the bag has filled.

My Occupational Therapy session ended at 9 o'clock with a wave goodbye and Joan's, "See you tomorrow morning." *Wait a minute. What about me?* Joan had left me lying on the bed wearing only my underwear, two socks and a pair of sweat pants around my ankles. Luckily I had a *full hour* to recover before I was scheduled to meet Hugh Simson in the 3 West Therapy Gym for PT.

I was exhausted, frustrated and—of course—hungry but I was determined not to let this small setback ruin the day. Summoning all my remaining strength, I reached back and pulled the call button to ring the nurses' station. "Can I help you?" was Unit Secretary Barbara Ford's quick response.

"Could you please ask my tech to come here," I asked, "I need help getting dressed."

A few minutes later, Ginny Wood, my day tech, came into the room, and seeing my predicament, could hardly contain her laughter. Her eyes teared, and little snorts emanated from her nose. But, being the professional that she was, Ginny kept her composure and went about the urgent business at hand.

Ginny helped me finish dressing, assisted me in using the slide board to get into my wheelchair, and wishing me a good morning sent me off to my physical therapy appointment like she might send a little boy off to a day at school.

I cruised past the nurses' station, waved to Barbara (a student pilot and fellow aviation enthusiast) and headed towards the skybridge. I'd decided to try out the new pair of leather-palmed Hatch gloves Hugh had recently given me. Gaining more confidence daily in controlling my wheelchair, I thought the slight downhill grade of the skybridge was an the ideal place to put on some speed and test how well I could slow down the wheelchair.

I gave the chair's wheels a couple of hefty tugs as I passed the Employee Lounge then entered the skybridge. My chair soon reached maximum velocity and I started to squeeze the wheel rims to slow it down, but the floor at the west end of the bridge dips so sharply, instead of slowing I picked up more speed! I squeezed the rims until I could feel the friction heat through my gloves, and then lightened my grip. My chair went still faster until suddenly the skybridge floor went uphill like a runaway truck ramp. Reacting as if it were in a field of sand, the chair slowed and I was able to make a sharp left but not before nearly mowing down Mark Gedman, another patient.

Mark was known all over Craig for his enthusiasm and upbeat spirit. (This translates to: he's a joker). He'd progressed in his rehabilitation from a wheelchair to walking with forearm crutches. *(See Chapter 14 for his story)* I congratulated Mark on his walking without assistance, and then used our chance meeting to ask him what he thought about the Therapy Pool. I knew Mark's affinity for water sports (his injury occurred while he was swimming). I asked him about the Therapy Pool where I had my first scheduled session later that day.

Mark laughed. "You mean you haven't seen it yet?" I answered that I hadn't. "You'd better be in good shape. The pool's kept hot and therapy is intense and non-stop."

Great! Just what I want to hear. I'm not even half-way through my first full day of rehab and I'm already bushed and my muscles screaming. I surmised my hour-long PT session with Hugh wasn't going to be easy. And I was right again!

PT started with Hugh showing me where the free weights and wall weights were kept. He advised me to use them every chance I could to strengthen my arms and upper body. Next, he instructed me on how to use a slide board to transfer from my wheelchair to the exercise mat. This turned out to be easy since the mat wasn't a floor mat; it was a large mat on a table that could be raised or lowered. Hugh lowered it for me so I could slide easily to the eight-foot square mat. After a few practice slides back and forth my PT class really shifted gears.

Lying on my back while Hugh manipulated my legs to stretch their muscles, I conjured up thoughts of the athletic trainers I had met during my younger days running track and playing hockey. Like then, I thought all I'd have to do was relax. I was wrong! Hugh took my right heel in one hand and, holding my right leg stiff near the knee with the other hand, lifted my leg to check the tightness of the hamstring muscles.

HOT DAMN! For someone who wasn't supposed to have any sensation below the waist I sure felt that! A sudden, sharp pain! My muscles were so tight Hugh could have played them like guitar strings.

Using all the upper body strength I could muster, I rolled over on my stomach then grimaced as Hugh abused my legs some more. (A pinched nerve caused some additional pain in my right hip and added to the discomfort.) I was amazed at how much my muscles had tightened in the short time I had been hospitalized.

The hour passed rapidly and when it was over I used the slide board to transfer from the mat back into my wheelchair and wheeled over to the water fountain to re-fill my now empty water bottle. Living in Colorado's high altitude, I learned it's essential to drink plenty of water every day. Add to that, the fact that I was undergoing strenuous physical exercise while draining urine continuously through the Foley Catheter, meant I needed to drink even more water.

I always carried a bottle with me wherever I went at Craig, usually in my lap or in the backpack hanging on the back of the wheelchair. There were plastic bottle holders that I could clamp on to the front frame bar of my wheelchair but I stopped using them because they protruded too far from the wheelchair and, if I got too close to a wall or doorway, they would hit it and break off.

It's interesting to note how little space there really is between a doorframe and a moving wheelchair or between a wheelchair and the bottom of a table or desk or any other inanimate object that kept getting in my way.

The PT session over, I wheeled back to my room to relax before lunch and to get ready for the afternoon's rehab. My tech Ginny came by again to see how I was doing. She evidently thought I was as beat as I felt, because she offered to bring lunch to my room rather than make me go back to the 3West cafeteria to get it.

Let me tell you, lunch in my room rarely happened. Not being one to turn down a generous offer, I agreed and soon was enjoying a meal of homemade bacon and tomato soup, almond chicken and rice casserole (with oriental mixed vegetables). This was topped off with strawberry Napoleon for dessert. I couldn't say whether the food was as good as it seemed or whether I was too hungry to think otherwise.

My afternoon schedule listed an education class at 1:00pm and my first PT class in the Therapy Pool at 2:30. I thought that, since the Education Classroom was right across from my room, I'd come back to my room between sessions to put on my bathing suit and then wheel down to the pool. Ginny didn't agree with my plan. (Remember, she'd already seen my attempt to dress myself).

"You'll need at least an hour to undress and dress again," she said. If I'm busy with another patient and you need my help, there's no way you'll get to the pool on time." She had a solution though.

She would help me change into my bathing suit right after lunch and I would attend the education class wearing a bathing suit under my sweat pants. This not only worked well that day, it became my standard routine whenever I was scheduled for pool PT after education classes.

I sat through my education class, "Spinal Cord Injury (SCI) Anatomy and Physiology" but only managed to stay awake after the terrific lunch by doing constant weight shifts in my wheelchair. Afterward, I wheeled across the skybridge to 3West and took the freight elevator to the first floor. There, I pulled right out of the elevator and into the Therapy Pool area.

The room holding the pool was constructed out of white brick and bordered with blue tile. The pool was not large as swimming pools go, but much larger than I thought it would be. It's kept at around ninety-five degrees to keep the pool chemicals stabilized. The pool has a five-foot deep end and a four-foot shallow end. At the shallow end there's a wide seven-step staircase with three handrails. Scattered around the pool were various rehab aids such as flotation devices, tubes, and ankle, foot and waist weights. The hallway wall is all windows so anyone can stop and watch. Despite the high temperature of the water and the room there was very little chemical odor noticeable.

Entering the pool area, I was greeted by Registered Physical Therapist (RPT) Carol Aikin, the aquatic therapy specialist. She directed me to place my wheelchair under a Guldmann Lift near the edge of the pool. Carol's volunteer assistant, Amanda Vargo, then helped me take off my sneakers, socks, shirt, and sweatpants. She put them in my wheelchair backpack and proceeded to put the lift's sling around my back and shoulders and under my thighs.

While waiting for Carol to get into the pool to receive me in the lift, I started chatting with Amanda and was surprised to learn that she was a Craig graduate. Having suffered a brain injury a few years earlier she now volunteered one day a week at the pool as a show of support for Craig. (*See Chapter 14 for Amanda's story*)

With Amanda standing next to my wheelchair looking on, Carol pushed the button on the lift controls and I slowly rose up out of the wheelchair, and, hanging like a side of beef on a conveyor belt, I was hoisted away from the chair, past the pool's edge, and suspended over the shallow end of the pool. Carol pushed another button and the miniature "Willy" (me) was lowered, butt first, into the ninety-four degree water.

I held on to the edge of the pool while the sling was removed and found myself actually standing up in the water. This was the first time I had been able to stand in three weeks and, even though I had no feeling in my legs or feet, it felt invigorating to be able to stretch my lower back and leg muscles.

Carol pointed to a bench that was in the water near me and said, "I want you to go sit on that, please."

I tried to walk to it but it was impossible to either move my legs or support my weight on them. I reached the bench by pulling myself along the poolside with my arms. Once there, I sat enjoying the warm water until Carol came over and strapped a pound and a half weight on each of my ankles.

Carol then demonstrated a series of leg exercises for me to do in the water to help strengthen my leg muscles. I listened but was thinking, *A lot of good her directions are going to do me. How can I exercise my legs if I can't move them?*—But, I could move my legs!

Using muscles I didn't know I had—and that didn't work well out of water—I managed to lift my feet just enough to get them off the floor of the pool to do some of the exercises. I was amazed at what I could do in water that I couldn't even think of doing out of the water.

For the next forty minutes I tried to walk, performed water exercises (not water ballet) and worked on other movements to increase my range of motion and stretch my muscles. Because of the resistance of the water it is difficult to fall and easy to remain upright. This gave me the opportunity to lift my legs (one at a time) and to flex my arms and hips, things I could not do in the gym. At all times, both Carol and Amanda held one of my arms to help me keep my balance which, to say the least, was non-existent. However, it sure felt good to have a woman on each arm. Too bad no one was there to see it.

My friend Mark Gedman (the guy I almost ran over with my wheelchair) was right on when he told me how intense pool therapy was. I felt good and strong after the session—but that would soon change.

Carol strapped me into the sling again and I was lifted out of the water, swung close to the edge of the pool and, while hanging there, Amanda hosed me down with warm water to remove as much of the pool chemicals as possible. After my unexpected shower, I was gently lowered back on to the wheelchair that Amanda had covered with white towels and a white, cotton blanket while I was in the pool.

After Amanda released me from the sling harness, she folded the blanket around me and filled in with some more towels, leaving me looking like Moby Dick with arms.

Wrapped up like a white whale gift package to keep me warm and dry and mustering the last bit of strength left in my arms, I wheeled my way back to the elevator, rode up to the third floor, and somehow made it across the skybridge back to my room. Once there, I turned the wheelchair around facing the door, and just sat there for twenty minutes as the sun went down outside.

Totally drained yet feeling warm and peaceful, I could have fallen asleep right in my chair, but my evening tech, Debbie, had seen me go in my room. She stopped by to help me get out of my blanket and my collection of towels, dress and make sure I had a dinner menu.

An important element of rehab at Craig is the staff's polite, but firm insistence that meals be eaten in one of the cafeterias and not in your room. This would have been easier for me if a cafeteria was closer but it was not. My choice was to go to the 3West gym where the corner of the PT area became a satellite cafeteria during meals or go to the Craig Cafeteria in the basement. Besides, I wanted to talk to Mark so I opted for the 3West gym where I knew he would be having dinner.

I put on my gloves again then forced my aching shoulder muscles to heave me and my chair back across the bridge and into the gym where two long tables had been set up next to the work out mats. Mark was already there, and so was my favorite younger patient Courtney Ferrall.

I wheeled up to the counter, pulled a tray from the rack and perused the evening's dinner choices—beef and bean burritos with green chili or a barbeque beef sandwich. Neither being a great favorite of mine I ordered the sandwich, some watermelon and a Sierra Mist to drink.

Leaving my tray on the counter, I wheeled my way over to where Mark was sitting and then parked my chair across from him. Jess, the food service assistant, carried my tray over to me.

Mark could tell right away that I had been through Carol's pool initiation. He gave me the expected "I told you so" look and started to heckle me but Mike's arrival spared me.

Mike, a quadriplegic from Wisconsin and a die-hard Green Bay Packer fan, drove up to our table in his power chair. He had been injured when he fell out of a tree stand while hunting resulting in paralysis from the neck down.

A good-natured man in his fifties, Mike had progressed to the point where he had regained some strength and upper body movement, and, using a special brace on his hand, could feed himself. His biggest complaint was always that his room was too cold. I thought maybe he was just a typical Packer fan who wanted an excuse to wear his green and yellow Packer sweatshirt. I'm not so sure if Denver Bronco fans are any less enthusiastic. When asked what he thought of pool therapy, Mike said he liked it a lot, mainly because the pool water was so warm.

I finished my meal then returned to my room to relax and to check the schedule to see what was on tap for the next day. It looked like a busy morning awaited me starting with an hour of "on the mat" with my physical therapist Hugh then an hour of exercises in the gym with PT Heather Stewart. My last morning class was at 11 o'clock, the schedule simply said, "Wheelchair Class" in the main gym.

Sounds like an easy way to wind up the morning. I liked the idea of sitting around getting lectured on how to properly use my manual wheelchair. Wrong again!

The next day's session with Hugh turned out as expected as he put me through a series of leg stretches that seemed to loosen up my tight leg muscles (but not enough to give me any real improved ability to move my legs without assistance.) Heather Stewart turned out to be a very quiet physical therapist who continued the same type of exercises that Hugh had done the previous hour.

I was beginning to feel relaxed as Heather held my ankles and worked my dormant leg muscles through a series of stretches. I started to worry I would become too relaxed to stay awake in my wheelchair class the next hour. I shouldn't have worried.

After Heather was finished with me, I wheeled myself to the elevator for the ride down to the west building first floor and then to the main gym. Wheeling down the hallway and eventually around the final corner, I came to a steep down-hill section of the hall that was actually a wide ramp. Cruising down the ramp, I slowed the chair with my gloved hands and swung it to the right and darted through the open gym door.

To my surprise Heather was already there and was working with John Minden, the RPT in charge, installing a set of long, temporary "tipper bars" on the lower back of a patient's wheelchair. (These bars prevent the chair from tipping over backwards during wheelchair exercises.)

I started to move towards the seating area on the sidewall of the gym when Heather spied me and called me over to where she and John were standing. "What size bars do you use?" she asked me. "I don't know. I've never been to this class before." Heather grinned, then, eyeing my chair said, "Let's try a 23."

Not having a clue as to what she was talking about, I nodded approval and waited while the two bars were quickly installed on my chair. As soon as she finished, John glared at me and said, "Well, don't just sit there. This is a wheelchair class. Start wheeling."

Again, I was clueless. Seeing my perplexed look, John asked, "First time?" I nodded. He smiled and said, "Every time you come to this class, have your tipper bars installed then wheel four laps around the gym, two forwards and two backwards." *Yeah right!* I thought. *I get plenty of exercise wheeling around...without this.*

I was less than thrilled with the prospect of training for the Wheelchair Olympics. However, never being one to resist authority (especially when authority is staring right at you) I grudgingly set out to make my laps. Four or five other patients zipped past me as though I was stuck in mud, but, slow or not, I was determined to complete the assigned laps.

Then it hit me. All the other patients in class were young enough to be my grandchildren. *Why bother trying to keep up with them? They're all a bunch of kids!* With these thoughts clouding my brain, I decided to slow down. Maybe John wouldn't notice how many laps I hadn't done.

Lost in thought I ambled one forward lap around the gym then turned the chair around to begin my backwards laps. All of a sudden Heather sped past me in a wheelchair and yelled, "Hurry it up, slowpoke." She then called everyone to the center of the gym floor for a demonstration on the proper way to do "wheelies."

I hadn't done wheelies since the fifties, and never in a wheelchair, so this was going to be interesting. Heather showed us how to tilt our chairs backwards so the front wheels are off the ground and our center of gravity was just behind the seat of our chairs. When done properly you can hold this position indefinitely. The question was, "Why?"

Of course, I couldn't get the hang of wheelies for anything despite trying over and over to get it. I eventually got to the point where I could get the front wheels up but I just couldn't get the feel for where my center of gravity was located. So while everyone—Heather included—did "wheelies," I was relegated to hanging in the back of the gym under the basketball net, to practice, practice, practice. This reminded me a little too much of my junior high gym classes.

I'll admit I liked other education classes at Craig far more than the wheelchair classes, but I sure grew to appreciate what handling a manual wheelchair entailed. I had to practice going up and down curbs, across streets, maneuvering in snow and ice and my favorite thing, going up and down stairs in a wheelchair.

Okay, you shouldn't go up the stairs alone but you can instruct others in how to assist you in moving the chair up or down, one step at a time, without getting jarred or dumped overboard. This enables you to use stairs when no ramps or elevators are available.

I'll confess, at least two days a week I skipped John's class—endurance run and game days. My TM had wiped out any endurance I had but that wasn't confirmed until I fumbled through a couple of endurance wheelchair classes.

My first try at one of these classes came after a group of us had been practicing going in and out of the hospital's doors. The eight other patients and three physical therapists, wearing ski jackets to keep warm in the Denver winter air, formed a line of wheelchairs to tour the streets of Englewood.

In short order I was last in the pack and soon the gap between me and the other wheelers kept increasing as the much younger patients went faster and faster. After a few more minutes, the group was out of sight so I decided to "forget it" and return to Craig. I was cold and my wheelchair gloves were not designed for winter use.

I turned my chair around and immediately realized that I had no idea where Craig or I was. Not being familiar at all with the area, all I could do was wheel to the nearest intersection and look around. On a light pole near the intersection was a blue and white "Hospital" sign that pointed up the street. *That's it, I guess.*

I decided that, since Swedish and Craig were the only two hospitals in the immediate area, I would go in the direction of the sign.

Deciding and "doing" soon became different things. The street to Craig went uphill at such a sharp angle that even able-bodied walkers were struggling and winded. There was no possible way I was going to get my wheelchair up that hill!

As I sat there pondering my dilemma, Audrey Natale, one of the PTs from the class came back on foot in search of a stray student…me. I explained, "I just couldn't keep up with those youngsters, so I stopped."

"You did the right thing," Audrey said, "But why are you going the long, difficult way?"

I shrugged. Audrey swung my chair around and aimed me in the opposite direction of the way the Hospital sign pointed. We traveled for about two hundred feet and went through a small alley. Emerging a block away, I could see Swedish Hospital only two easy blocks from me, with Craig another block from there. That's when I learned about the connecting areas between Swedish and Craig.

Instead of going straight to Craig, we went in the main entrance of Swedish, down a corridor to what looked like a tunnel and came out in the basement of Craig's west building. And that was my first try at a wheelchair endurance class. It was nice to get outside for some fresh air…I guess.

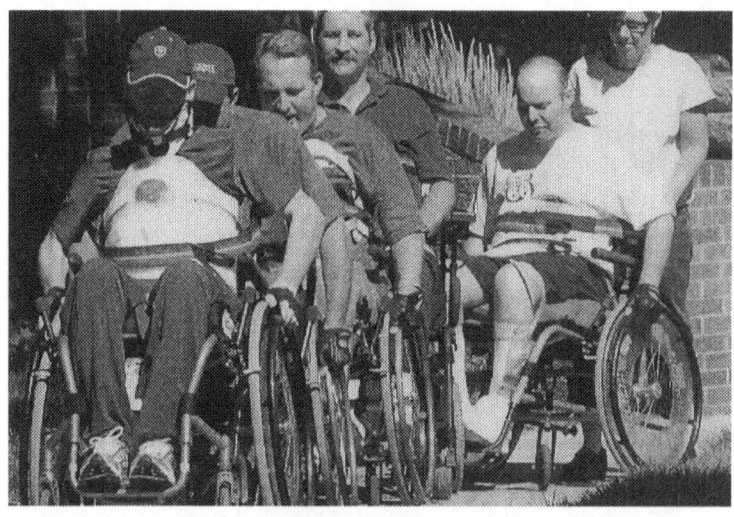

Endurance Run   Fig. 5–3

My second try at the endurance class came a week later when Jill was visiting me. She decided to walk along while the class wheeled. We all left the gym and went in the same direction as the previous week and, like the previous week, the class left me in the dust. (or was it snow?)

After twenty minutes of puffing and straining to keep up, I threw in the towel. Luckily Jill was with me and I remembered where Craig was so we just turned around and cut the class short.

Game day was another of the class days I elected to skip...after I tried it once, which was enough. My first Friday morning after moving to the east building I had arrived right on time for the usual eleven o'clock Wheelchair Class. I noticed there were several more patients than usual attending and most of the male patients (all paraplegics), were wearing shorts rather than sweat pants. Some had on brightly colored headbands. Those headbands should have been clue enough for me to hightail it out of the gym.

Yikes! Look out!

John announced, "Today is Go Ball. Let's pick teams."

Rusty, a teenager I'd met in the cafeteria earlier told me the rules. The goal of the game was to carry a small, football-like ball down the length of the gym in your chair then throw it into the goal for a score. You had to pass the ball to a free teammate, as the opposing team would try to block you from moving towards the goal. *Okay, sounds easy.*

Go Ball sounded easy but turned out to make the movie *Murderball* look as tame as a Disney feature. I was picked to be a player on Rusty's team. The other team was short two players so (PT) Heather and Rusty's father Alvin, (Yes, Rusty's father. Friends and family are encouraged to participate in all phases of rehabilitation) grabbed wheelchairs and the game was on.

Right after the game started I caught a long throw by a teammate then started towards the goal, but my progress stopped when I was surrounded by players from the other team. Just as they closed in on me, I threw the ball to Rusty who proceeded to haul down the floor towards the goal.

An opposing player blocked Rusty by ramming him at an angle going full speed, and catapulted him out of his restraining straps and his chair to land spread eagled on the gym floor. Rusty didn't even wait a second for help to arrive. He flipped himself over and pulling himself along the floor with tremendous arm strength and bleeding from cuts to his knuckles, he reached his chair and tried to pull himself up. By then, assistance came from the bench and he was hoisted back into his chair and sent back into the game.

I lasted about two minutes and, after realizing that this "so-called" sport had too much contact for me, I retired to the sidelines. I decided I'd leave the game to the youngsters, unless, of course, there was protective gear available.

Heading back upstairs to the third floor gym to do some weight therapy, I bumped into Hugh who happened to be on his way downstairs to find me. He told me it was time I was fitted for and trained to use a power wheelchair, because, as he explained, it was assumed that I would not improve beyond where I was at that moment and, if I did not improve, I would definitely need a power chair rather than a manual chair, especially to go longer distances than a block or two. Hugh and I went to the 3West gym where I quickly learned how to transfer from chair to chair and found myself excited to start using a power chair. It looked easy to operate and the thought of not having to wear gloves anymore or exert so much energy getting myself around was simply overwhelming. I had wheels.

6

Occupational Therapy: Frustration & Fun

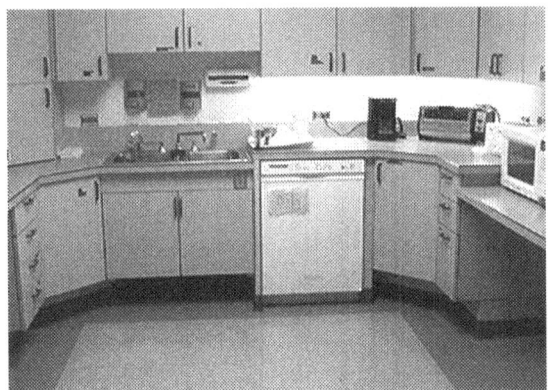

Fig. 6–1

While physical therapy is concerned with getting your body to function as well as possible, occupational therapy is concerned with helping you learn, or re-learn, how to do the everyday, normal activities that you used to do without thinking. OT emphasizes self-sufficiency and independence in dressing, bathing, attending to personal hygiene and other personal tasks as well as cooking, cleaning, doing laundry and other household tasks.

Occupational Therapy played a crucial role in my overall recovery plan and was intertwined with all other disciplines of my rehabilitation plan. The OTs worked closely with the PTs to schedule patients and conduct all aspects of the program. My OTs usually had me doing things that were difficult, different, and usually rewarding.

After my primary Occupational Therapist, Donna, finished my first day of testing and after the anguish of trying to dress myself under the watchful eye of

OT Joan, I became the permanent project of Certified Occupational Therapist Assistant (COTA), Dana Lee. For the next six weeks she pushed, cajoled, pleaded, ordered, demanded and did whatever else it took (including threatening) to get me to the point of independence and self-sufficiency.

Dana knew when to push me and when to back off, when to praise my efforts and when to laugh at my shortcomings, when I was feeling strong enough to last a little longer, and when I was in pain and should stop what I was doing. Of course, she was in cahoots (they call it communication) with my physical therapist Hugh. Somehow, someway she seemed to always know exactly what he'd done with me the hour before she had her turn with me.

One morning after a particularly grueling PT session with Hugh in the 3West gym, I was happy my next class with Dana was scheduled to be right there in the gym. I thought I'd probably just do some light stretches on the mat or other exercises that wouldn't be too strenuous.

Right at ten o'clock Dana marched out of the OT office, checked my Foley leg bag to see if it needed draining, then said, "Follow me!"

Dana did an about face and walked twenty feet to a small room located next to the food service window just off the gym. I wheeled in behind her and saw the room was a fully equipped kitchen complete with sink, stove, oven, microwave, toaster and many more appliances and kitchen gadgets. There was nobody cooking or baking so the kitchen was mine for an hour. (I suspect this was the way Dana had planned it.)

I turned to Dana and asked: "What am I cooking today?"

"Nothing," she replied, "You're not ready to cook just yet. Let's wait to see how well you progress with other things…like *cleaning*, for instance."

Before I could react, Dana opened a box of oatmeal and dumped a couple of hands full of it, plus some tissue scraps, on the floor. Turning to me, she handed me a straw broom and dustpan. "I want you to do just what you would at home to clean this up. I want to see how well you function in that wheelchair." I looked at the mess on the floor. *This is not what I had in mind for this morning.*

"I'm going to my office for a second to get some evaluation forms," Dana said. "Go ahead and do exactly what you would do at home to clean up this spill."

Three minutes later, Dana returned to find me sitting in the exact same position I'd been in when she had left me. The oatmeal was in the same position too. Looking a little perplexed, she asked, "What's wrong? Why haven't you even started using the broom and dustpan?"

"You told me to do exactly what I would do at home in these circumstances, and I did."

Then, without even cracking a smile, I said, "I called Housekeeping and they'll be here within the hour!" So there!

After Dana stopped laughing, she drove me hard to pick up every single flake of dried oatmeal and tissue scrap. This was done by wheeling over to the oatmeal or tissue, bending over and, using the broom, sweeping the oatmeal into the dustpan, then wheeling over to the trash bin and dumping it.

The laugh we shared was the start of a special relationship of mutual respect and understanding that soon developed for me into a feeling of trust. I no longer questioned what she did but tried my best to not only accomplish every task she gave me, but to excel beyond both of our aims. Knowing this, I suspect Dana strove to keep raising the bar to see if I could follow. To tell the truth, the way I still feel about Dana, I think I would follow her anywhere! And believe me, she led me all over the place.

A week after the kitchen duty, Dana announced that the next morning's OT session would be held in my room instead of the gym. Anticipating another dressing session, I expertly hid the most difficult to put on clothing and neatly laid out the best sweat pants and T-shirt that I could find. But, much to my dismay, Dana entered the room with a large vacuum cleaner and an even larger smile. I let out a big sigh. Sensing my letdown, Dana said, "Well at least this time I didn't bring any tissues or oatmeal."

The bedroom half of the suite and the bathroom had a tile floor so I didn't vacuum there but the other half was carpeted. It didn't take me long to clean it, even in my wheelchair.

Then, without so much as giving me a break, Dana pushed the vacuum cleaner out the door, and called back to me, "Let's go!"

Out the door I went, trying to catch up with her as she walked rapidly towards the skybridge and over to 3 West—and the gym. I never even came close to catching up to her because when I wheeled past the nurses' station I noticed that the lunch menus were there, so naturally, I stopped to take one.

When I finally arrived at the gym Dana was already waiting there with Hugh and Ken Russo, the wheelchair specialist, and a demo model Quickie power wheelchair. The power chair was for me to use for a few days to see if I liked it. (Due to insurance restrictions, I couldn't have both a manual and a power chair. If my condition didn't improve, a power chair would be a necessity.)

Dana and Ken worked on fitting the power chair to my body: adjusting the seat height, braking affect and general overall structure and workings, while Hugh proceeded to put me through some exercises to strengthen my legs and then some other muscle tightening exercises designed to keep my paralyzed bladder muscles from permanent damage. I finally had enough of the exercises and decided to try out the new chair.

Using the slide board, I transferred from the mat into the power chair. My seat cushion had already been removed from the manual chair and placed on the power chair.

The Quickie power chair was higher than the manual chair and much, much heavier. Since it was controlled by a single toggle switch placed at the front of the right armrest, all I had to do was engage my thumb and forefinger and away I went. Using a method similar to one used to program a TV or VCR, Dana had programmed the chair to keep it fairly slow. I felt confident that I was in good hands and that it shouldn't be difficult to operate the power chair.

After I did a few practice turns, including sharp 180° left and right turns, Dana said, "Let's go see how fast that thing is."

We left the gym with Dana leading the way, and headed to the third floor elevator bank and took the elevator to the basement. Exiting the elevator, we went right and down the corridor to the tunnel that leads to Swedish Medical Center.

There wasn't a soul in the corridor so Dana said, "Just aim the chair down the hallway and hold the toggle switch in a straight forward position."

Feeling a little bit tentative, I maneuvered the chair to the centerline of the corridor and readied for takeoff. I expected a surge of raw power would take the chair, with me in it, to the edge of the sound barrier.

Instead, I soared down the corridor at approximately 5–6 miles an hour, (much faster than a manual wheelchair but not exactly a Chuck Yeager feat.)

At the end of the corridor, I slowed down and repeated my effort in the reverse direction. Dana was waiting, clearly amused. "I'm glad my programming to slow the speed worked. I'm sure you would have liked to have gone faster but, for obvious safety reasons, I can't permit it."

Seeing that I could comfortably maneuver this new power chair, Dana decided to let me find out how good I was in light snow and on a ramp. Turning slightly to the right of where we were standing, we came to the cafeteria and the door to the patio area. I'd gone through this door with my manual chair many times so going through it with the power chair was a breeze. It only took a few minutes of me driving the chair down and back up the small snow-covered ramp near the patio to convince Dana I would be safe using the chair without supervision.

Of course, that's when Murphy's Law came into play.

Planning to return to the building through the mostly empty cafeteria (it was in between mealtimes), I started to go in through the patio door but couldn't quite hold the door open wide enough with one arm and operate the toggle switch at the same time. (Dana, meanwhile, stood mute behind me, observing how I would handle a situation like this.) I must have looked like a spastic juggler.

After finally figuring out how to alternate between pushing the door open with my left hand and controlling the chair with my right hand, I zoomed through the door into the cafeteria and headed straight for an empty table sitting only four or five feet away from me. Without any hesitation, I lifted my hand from the toggle switch. That was supposed to trigger the chair's braking system, but it didn't work!

The power chair and I kept going, crashed head on into a chair, then a table and came to a stop. Luckily my footrest protected my toes and legs and nobody had been seated at the table. I knocked a piece of metal from the front of the footrest off. Did I activate the airbags?

Dana was visibly upset, yet laughing at the same time. "You should have been wearing a helmet and some protective gear."

Luckily, Wheelchair Repair and Maintenance was right down the hall from the cafeteria. It seems the snow had shorted out the wheelchair's brake system, but since this was a common occurrence, there were repair parts on hand. The chair was running again within minutes and I returned to the gym to retrieve my manual chair and ask for a tech to help me get both chairs back to my room.

It was my belief that PT was to put me in shape to withstand the rigors of OT but the overlap was so significant that sometimes I didn't know the difference between them.

As I progressed, Hugh would "sign off" on my room chart to allow me to do certain things unassisted and unobserved that I hadn't been permitted to do alone before. For example, he had to clear me to travel alone around the Craig Campus, to dress myself and to transfer myself from my wheelchair to the chair or couch in my suite.

One of the aspects of OT is teaching a patient, and his family, how to cope with real life situations—simple situations like shopping, cruising a mall, bowling, preparing a meal or even going to a movie. These things are easily handled by able-bodied people but can be daunting to a wheelchair bound person. At Craig both Occupational Therapy and Therapeutic Recreation, address potential problem areas in real life.

It was a few weeks before I learned what therapeutic recreation meant. I guessed this department provided the same services as OT and PT but in a more relaxed and informal setting. I knew Therapeutic Recreation also provided an area where patients could go to watch a wide screen TV, play checkers or chess and use one of the department's computers.

Craig's Therapeutic Recreation department (the largest hospital-based Therapeutic Recreation department, in terms of number of employees and dedicated facilities, in the country) provides key resources in the rehabilitation process by offering programs directly related to the patient's physical reintegration in the community, and maximizing the ability to enjoy various types of recreational options, plus discovering and exploiting hidden or little known artistic and other talents.

The "Rec" Department, as it's called by the patients, has a ceramics kiln, a large selection of art supplies and a greenhouse. It sponsors local outings in which a limited number of patients, accompanied by Rec and OT supervisors, learn to mingle and manage in crowds, enjoy a good movie at a theatre or go to a professional sporting event. These activities are designed not only to allow patients to relax but also to give them the knowledge and confidence to realize that they can do whatever they choose after they're discharged. It's for this reason patients are encouraged to participate in at least two outings.

Although many of its outings are "spectator" outings, the Rec department also sponsors "participation" outings. Joe Gomez, Director of Therapeutic Recreation, and his staff schedule and supervise popular outings including: bowling, white water rafting, scuba diving and hot air ballooning. Being a long-time balloon pilot myself, I was excited to think I would get a chance to fly again with pilots I was sure to have known previously. Because I was discharged from Craig prior to the next scheduled balloon outing, I never did get that chance.

The Rec department also hosts several parties throughout the year. Patients and staff celebrate everything from official holidays like Halloween and Christmas, to the athletic holidays like the Super Bowl. All patients are invited to attend and are expected to get to the Rec department on time and on their own when possible. (This creates some problems once in a while when there is a line of people at the second and third floor elevators waiting to get to the first floor Rec department.)

Just prior to the end of the month, a new Therapeutic Recreation Schedule, showing each day's activities for the coming month, is taped to all patients' room doors. The schedule lists all outings, in-house activities and volunteer activities planned for the coming month. As an example, the December 2004 schedule shows the following outings:

♦ Shopping at Wal-Mart

- Fast Food Dinner & Christmas Lights Tour

- Movie Theatre Outing

- NFL Broncos/Dolphins Game at Mile High Stadium

- Scuba Diving

- Colorado Eagles Hockey

- Museum & Imax

- "Taste of China" Buffet

- Shopping at Southglenn Mall

The TR staff also provided in-house activities such as: Christmas tree decorating, cooking classes, movie showings, ornament making, wheelchair tennis lessons, computer classes, horticulture, and arts and crafts.

Volunteers planned the balance of the activities. Their December list included guitar lessons, facials, manicures, pet therapy with two huge Newfoundland dogs, and a visit from the Denver Bronco Cheerleaders.

If a patient attended all the activities sponsored by Therapeutic Recreation, there would be no time left for OT, PT or anything else. Believe me, sometimes I was tempted.

In retrospect, it is clear that occupational therapy played an extremely important role in my rehabilitation by emphasizing the need to accomplish the routine tasks first. By doing this, the performance of routine tasks became automatic, evolving as the building blocks for performing more difficult tasks in the future.

7

The Medical Staff:
Leading the Rehab Team

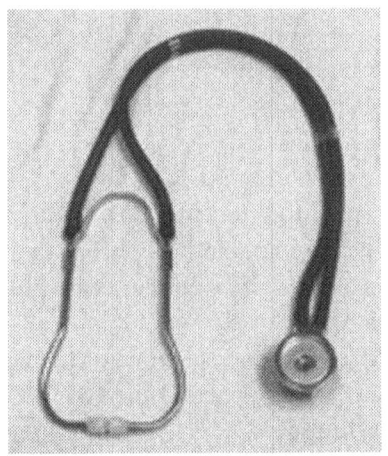

Fig. 7–1

Leading the entire rehab team is Craig's medical staff. My medical team members not only include my attending physician, nurses and techs but also consulting specialists and lab technicians. Craig has a working agreement with its next-door neighbor Swedish HealthONE Medical Center. In fact, the hospitals are linked together by a corridor in the basement of Craig's West Building and on Swedish's third floor.

The Craig Hospital-Swedish Hospital affiliation goes back several years. Swedish predates Craig by two years (1905 and 1907 respectively) and was originally a five-acre tuberculosis tent city sanatorium founded by Dr. Charles Bundsen.

Swedish is a first class medical facility that includes an around-the-clock Level I Trauma center complete with two often-used helicopter landing pads. It boasts a full complement of specialties such as surgery, neurology, orthopedics, pediatrics, radiology, and pathology. Craig patients receive specialized medical services from Swedish Hospital. Swedish physicians make rounds at both Swedish and Craig.

Not having to maintain a complete medical staff and facility, Craig's resources are better utilized for rehabilitation while at the same time, its patients receive the best medical attention possible without having their recovery disrupted by travel to other medical facilities.

Craig physicians are part of CNS Medical Group, PC, an independent company that has provided spinal cord and brain injury specialization to individuals at Craig Hospital since 1972.

Under the Craig Hospital team approach, one physician is assigned to each team and is assigned the role of team leader. My rehab team's leader (also my attending physician) was Dr. Shih-Fong Hsu, MD., a Physiatrist. (a doctor certified as a specialist in rehabilitative medicine specifically dedicated to diagnosis and treatment of physical disabilities.)

Every day, Dr. Hsu came to my room to review my progress with me. Our discussions were usually frank and forthcoming. We often considered my rehabilitation plan, my overall health status and any medication changes he was considering implementing. Once in a while we discussed the results of a lab test he'd ordered, a change in procedure or a change in my program.

My biggest concern was what permanent damage might result from my TM. Dr. Hsu's biggest concern was deciphering the possible correlation between the TM and my Parkinson's disease.

Even though I had daily contact with Dr. Hsu, it was usually the duty nurse—second in order of authority below the team leader—who actually filled me in on what his orders were. Most nurses worked a twelve-hour shift so I had only two nurses in each twenty-four hour period. The duty nurses were assigned five patients each for the shift and regularly scheduled nurses were usually responsible for the same patients. This way, the nurses could remain on a patient's team their entire stay at Craig. The day shift nurses, knowing their patients very well, represented the medical department at patient conferences.

All the nurses assigned to 3East were excellent, but I was fortunate to have had six *outstanding* nurses. Shelbi Raffelock, Peggy Hogan, Gerald McGinley and Debbie Shultz on the day shift and Lilia Smith and Kathy Kloczkowski on the night shift are extremely knowledgeable and professional but with distinct and separate personalities and work methods. Lilia and Kathy tended to be introspective and laid back, while Gerry, Shelbi, Peggy and Debbie tended to be more outgoing and hurried. Maybe it had something to do with the shifts they worked.

Every morning, the day shift nurses made a point to see each of their assigned patients before the patients left the floor for scheduled therapy or classes. Usually the nurses started their visits early (around 7:15am). Even though each nurse had only five patients to see, taking vital signs and administering injections and medications took time. Sometimes their routine was disrupted when attending physicians came in to review their patients' charts.

For some unknown reason, it seemed I was either first or last on my nurse's list, but never in between. I'm sure it had a lot to do with who my tech was on any given day. Most of them knew I liked to get dressed and into my wheelchair by seven o'clock. Tech Ginny Wood was especially diligent in making sure I was up and out.

During my first few weeks when I couldn't dress myself and still used a Foley Catheter, Ginny made sure I was the first patient seen by both her and the duty nurse. After I had progressed to the point of being able to dress myself, she'd stick her head through my doorway to make sure I was dressing. If I was doing fine, she'd say, "I'll be back in ten to help you into the wheelchair," and then, without fail, exactly ten minutes later I would hear her knock on the door.

Whenever I had my breakfast finished, Foley leg bag emptied and in place, wheelchair gloves on and five minutes left until my first scheduled activity, I just left my room...whether or not the duty nurse had been there with my medications. If the nurse happened to see me leave, I usually was told to wait. Then I had to go back to my room to await my Heparin shot (*referred to in Chapter 4*), seven or eight pills, a blood pressure cuff squeeze and a temperature probe in my ear.

Of course, escaping to the 3West gym or an education class offered only temporary escape from receiving my medications. Since prescribed medications and their timely use were essential to proper recovery, my nurses always finished with their patients still on 3East then hunted me down to give me mine.

More than once, Shelbi, Debbie or Peggy would intercept me in the gym or hallway and halt whatever I was doing to administer a shot to my gut and watch me down eight pills. Once in a while they remembered to bring a small container of applesauce from my refrigerator that I could take my pills with. (Shortly after moving to 3East, I discovered that putting all the pills into my applesauce made the process so much easier and the pills better tasting.)

As I stated, my four regularly scheduled, professional, confident and experienced day shift nurses had distinct personalities. Peggy had been a rehab nurse for

30 years and went about her business with speed and a no-nonsense attitude. She kept a straight face but had a great sense of humor behind it, and, like Shelbi and Debbie, liked to sit with me when things were quiet, and talk about any subject that happened to come up. I valued that.

I think one of the best facets of the Craig rehab philosophy is the way casual, open discourse between staff and staff, patient and patient and staff and patient is encouraged. I'd been hospitalized before, but had never been involved in the type of openness present at Craig.

Debbie, the quietest of the day shift nurses, was a tech for twelve years before becoming an RN. She then spent six years in the Cardiac Unit at Swedish before returning to Craig in 2000. She seemed a little reluctant at first to engage in small talk with me, but after a while she came by my room regularly and we had some thought-provoking discussions.

Debbie also had a terrific sense of humor. I had made some funny door signs on the computer, (*Doin' My Thing, Stay Out; In Conference, Come Back in Ten Minutes)* and she liked them so much, she asked me to make some signs for other patients.

Shelbi was definitely a no-nonsense nurse but went about the serious business of SCI nursing with a smile and a positive attitude. She had been a nurse only two years when I met her. (One of a growing number of women who go back to school after raising a family.) Sometimes her approach seemed gruff but I believe she was a personification of Craig's "No Whining" policy. Her patients really appreciated it.

Gerald "Gerry" McGinley had been a nurse at Craig for twenty-nine years, starting right out of nursing school. He'd seen Craig through lots of growth and expansion and experienced the changes in treatment philosophy and environment that is now Craig. His infectious laugh could be heard all through the hallways as he constantly injected humor into his work, especially when Barbara or Cindy was manning the desk or if any patient happened to be nearby. Gerry loved an audience and if a patient was looking for a tech, all he would have to do was follow the sound of laughter coming from the 3East nurses' station. In all probability a group of techs (especially close to shift change) including Alex, Jeff, Terry, Kristin, JJ or the two Jennifers would be Gerry's willing audience.

Cindy Hardinger had been at Craig for twenty-four years, was a Unit Secretary and had listened to Gerry's stories longer than anyone else. In addition to her three-year stint in the Research Department and managing the desk at every SCI and TBI unit at one time or another, Cindy was also a Craig graduate, being in a wheelchair since 1977. The first-year nurse who took care of Cindy as a patient in 1977? Gerry McGinley.

The night shift nurses, Kathy and Lilia, were as different as day and night, but as professional and capable as anyone could want. Kathy had been a nurse at Craig only two and a half years when I met her, and before that was a tech. When I first met Kathy, I must admit I thought she was a Candy Striper because she looked young enough to be a teenager. She was very pretty, strong and had a smile that could light up a room. Although she appeared young, her knowledge and demeanor convinced me she was just as capable and professional as any of the more experienced nurses.

Both Lilia and Kathy liked to visit me last on their evening rounds, that way we could talk at length without much interruption. Like the day shift nurses, we talked about every subject imaginable—from medicine to current events—and soon developed a mutual trust and understanding that went a long way in assisting me in my rehabilitation.

Lilia, the more experienced nurse of the two, had an unbelievable talent for explaining complex medical topics to less than medically inclined patients—like me. She explained in understandable language the details of each procedure I was scheduled to undergo (i.e. Cystogram, Cystoscopy) and any new medication I was prescribed to take.

Not only was Lilia knowledgeable, she never hesitated to use the computer at the nurses' station to download charts, graphs, illustrations and explanations for me. I learned to be ready for a complete answer whenever I asked a question. She was also a terrific teacher, as my IC story will illustrate.

After I'd been at Craig for two weeks, my day nurse, Peggy came to me in the morning, looked at my chart and said, "I see that Dr. Hsu entered an order today that says your Foley Catheter is to be removed and you are to go on IC." She explained that the risk of getting a urinary tract infection increased greatly the longer the catheter remained in place.

Looking at her with a surprised look on my face, I asked, "If the Foley is removed, how am I supposed to pee, and what's an IC?"

"The IC is how you are going to pee and it means Intermittent Catheterization."

"Oh, I understand. Instead of a full time catheter, you're going to catheterize me on a set schedule."

"The set schedule is correct," she said, "but you're going to catheterize yourself."

When her words hit me my face must have turned ashen. "I'm going to do what?"

"Don't worry, it's a simple procedure that you'll have down pat in no time."

Right. You're not the one who's going to…

Peggy told me that I would be taught the procedure for an IC Sterile Catheterization in a few days and would have the Foley removed after studying the technique required. Peggy left the room and returned a few minutes later with a single sheet of yellow paper that had a page and a half of instructions and diagrams on how to do a self-catheterization.

Now, for the first time since I had been hospitalized, I felt very uneasy. Needles didn't bother me, getting stitches didn't bother me, having blood drawn didn't bother me, but the thought of sticking a tube into my own penis and threading it through to my bladder BOTHERED ME!

After two days of plotting every excuse known to mankind to try to get out of "this situation," I reluctantly began to accept the inevitable. I decided to quiz other patients about their experience with self-catheterization. Carefully choosing patients who had been at Craig the longest, (they tended to be much more open to discussions about things like this), I asked my questions.

Everyone had a different experience. Some had a lot of trouble with the procedure and some just took it in stride. I was surprised to learn that even the female patients were taught IC procedures. Somewhat reassured, I was beginning to feel a little better and was glad I still had a few days to reread the instructions. Fooled again!

At four o'clock that afternoon, Shelbi came into my room and asked me to get on my bed. She was there to remove my Foley. Reluctantly, I transferred onto the bed whereby Shelbi helped me pull down my sweat pants and then swiftly and painlessly removed the catheter.

That evening after meds were handed out, Lilia came into my room carrying a large box that she took into the bathroom. She came out holding a tray wrapped in clear plastic, pulled up a chair next to my bed and said, "I will do this procedure the first time if you like and then watch you as many times as it takes until I am sure you are comfortable doing it yourself."

I don't know where my bravado came from, but I told her that I had read the instructions many times and was sure, with her guidance, I could do it myself the first try.

"OK, if you're sure, lets do it," Lilia said. She handed me the tray and some packaged towelettes. After I cleaned my hands, Lilia and I proceeded to go through the instructions item by item. Lilia precisely explained how and why each step was done and the importance of following the steps in the order they're given.

Sitting up in my bed, I put on the sterile gloves, placed the required items in the sterile tray and draped the small sterile cloth (included in the kit) over my thighs. All went well until the time came to insert the catheter, which is simply a narrow tube about sixteen inches long—it looked more like a garden hose at the time. My body, sensing what was about to happen and ignoring my attempt at self-assurance, went into a defensive posture. This is difficult to explain but George Costanza's "shrinkage" on that famous episode of *Seinfeld* was nothing compared to mine.

Seeing how nervous I'd become, Lilia explained that there should be little or no feeling but, if I felt any discomfort, a small infusion of Lidocaine (topical anesthetic) would numb me.

I proceeded slowly, felt no discomfort. "How will I know when this thing reaches my bladder"? (I had visions of pushing the catheter through my bladder and into my liver.)

Lilia just nodded and said, "You'll know. Just go slowly, a couple of inches at a time."

I proceeded as Lilia directed. Suddenly my bladder started emptying through the catheter into the bag attached to the other end. When my bladder was empty, the flow suddenly stopped and I removed the catheter, easily without any pain or discomfort. Lilia smiled knowingly and said, "I told you so. Look how you got upset for nothing. I've been teaching this for years and everyone is surprised at how easy it is."

Was she ever right. Lilia told me that I did so well she was going to let me do it alone four hours later. She would come in after I was finished to check on me. Sure enough, the night tech, JJ, woke me up at one o'clock and I proceeded to catheterize (cath) myself without a hitch and called for Lilia to tell her. She said to keep a log of the amount drained each time, and that because of the amount that drained the first two times, I could cath every six hours instead of every four.

I told Lilia what a great teacher she was and then, feeling total relief, turned out the lights and went to sleep.

My rehab team consisting of Dr. Hsu, the nurses, and the techs, etc., received support from other medical specialists such as a neurologist, urologist, hematologist, radiologist and a manipulative therapist.

The neurologist, Dr. Cilo, monitored the advance of my Parkinson's and made sure the medication I was taking for it was effective without interfering with my rehabilitation. I only saw Dr. Cilo a couple of times but each time I was impressed with his knowledge and took his suggestions seriously.

The hematologist was Dr. Raul Alvarez. I spoke with him on a regular basis because TM cases are few and far between and he wanted to see if, through various blood tests, he could positively confirm the TM diagnosis and, more importantly, find the cause. In addition to TM I had a condition known as Polycythemia that, in plain terms, means I have too many red blood cells (high hematocrit) and too much blood. It's not severe and can be monitored through monthly blood tests. If the test shows my hematocrit count is elevated, the treatment is to simply drain off a few hundred ccs of blood. However, between the two conditions, Dr. Alvarez was constantly ordering different blood tests.

Having these tests gave me the chance to get to know one of the silent yet supporting members of the rehab team, Dominic Ziccardi. Dominic was a lab technician at Swedish Medical Center but did the lab work for Craig. He started his "bloodletting" early in the morning and always came to my room carrying a large tray filled with glass tubes sporting various colored tops.

Always polite, Dominic would say, "Good morning Mr. Tabak, I'm here again to draw some blood. Just two this time." He filled fourteen vials of blood the first time he visited. After that, he was always quick to let me know it was only one or two that he needed.

After finding out Dominic and I were both originally from the New York City area and baseball fans, seeing him became less of a nuisance and more of a pleasure.

Dominic was so good at what he did, so good, in fact, that one time when he came to draw some blood we started talking about the Yankees and George Steinbrenner. After a while, I finally asked, "When are you going to draw my blood?"

"I'm finished." Dominic answered. He had poked me and drawn the blood and I hadn't even felt it or noticed him doing it.

Some members of my rehab team were like ghosts. I felt their presence but never met them. Most of these people were the night shift techs and techs in training. I also rarely saw the techs that worked the eleven to seven o'clock night shift.

The first tech assigned to me the night I transferred to 3East from 3West, was Debbie Arellano, who alternated between the day and evening shifts. She had been a tech for two years and not only knew her stuff but went about her work with efficiency and a smile. She couldn't help but broadcast a great sense of humor. Her only shortcoming though, is her devotion to her patients.

Debbie would stay with a patient who wanted to talk to her, even if doing so would monopolize her time and drag her behind schedule. This devotion was great—when you were the one she was letting talk. Otherwise, you had to resign yourself to waiting at least an hour past your scheduled time with her. When Debbie was on duty and I knew I was going to need her assistance with dressing or my evening program, etc., I just scheduled to see her an hour prior to the time I really wanted her.

Stephanie Ball, another evening tech, was Debbie's opposite—rarely even a few minutes late. If she was supposed to meet me in my room at seven o'clock, she was in my room at seven o'clock. Stephanie had only been at Craig for a little over a year but she exuded the confidence that comes with many years of experience.

I was just starting to see some positive results from my rehabilitation when I became Stephanie's patient. Her first night with me had a full schedule that included helping me get undressed, transferring me out of my wheelchair onto a commode chair, assisting with my evening program, wheeling me to the shower, wheeling me out of the shower and assisting me in transferring from the commode chair back to my bed.

The commode chair is like a huge wheelchair but rather than a solid seat, it has an open bottom cushioned seat and wheels right over the top of a toilet. I used this chair so I could effectively complete my nightly bowel program. After completing the program, the chair was easily moved from the toilet area to the bathroom's shower area. I used the commode chair until shortly before my discharge, when I found I could maneuver to the bathroom without assistance and instead use a padded, standing commode chair.

Some of the night techs that I had only cursory knowledge of came into my room every two hours during the night to turn me. They needed to turn me to prevent me from getting bedsores that could possibly develop into infections that could prove fatal.

Getting turned while I slept was extremely annoying, though. (Who wants to wake up this way?) From the very beginning of my stay at Craig, I had excellent upper body strength, so besides being able to pull myself up towards the head of the bed, I was able to turn my body, thus eliminating the need for help with this.

As I progressed in my rehabilitation and finally reached a point where I could stand and walk, albeit gingerly, I found that I also could also turn myself in bed without any assistance. In my mind, this obviated the need for techs to come in and turn me, but I couldn't convince them of this. Their nocturnal turning finally got so aggravating that I complained about it to my duty nurse. I told her

I wasn't getting any sleep and asked would she get Dr. Hsu to write an order stopping it.

Somehow this plea reached the right person and all at once the body turning stopped and I was able to sleep uninterrupted. Yes!

There was also another procedure that tended to wake me up during the night too. Before I was able to stand the techs needed to monitor my possible muscle deterioration. Using a cloth measuring tape similar to those tailors or dressmakers use, they measured changes in my calf muscle size and upper and lower thigh muscle size. They did this two or three times a week.

The problem with measuring was they would wake me up in the middle of the night to do it. "Why" I asked, "Can't you do this when I'm being turned?" No answer. Later on when I started doing IC during the night, they still woke me up at another time to measure me. "Can't you do this after I do IC?" Again, no answer, and I never did get one, but, during my last two weeks at Craig, I was never bothered when I was sleeping.

An adjunct to Craig Hospital's regular medical services are non-traditional and supporting type services. These services include acupuncture, manipulative therapy, dental care and eye care.

Due to my Parkinson's and a sciatic nerve problem, I was scheduled for therapy with Craig consultant, Beverly Parrott, who saw patients two days a week on 2East.

Beverly is nationally known and has been a physical therapist since 1966. Her treatments were painful at first, but they allowed me to be relatively pain free afterwards. She was extremely knowledgeable and explained my afflictions and their suggested treatment in great detail. (Although I really didn't want to know about all the little things I had somehow acquired by getting older such as spinal deterioration, it was reassuring to find out that, for the most part, they were a normal part of the aging process and easily treated.)

Beverly's assistant, Massage Therapist Jane Meads, also helped ease my pain by administering Ultrasound treatments at the end of each session. She also gave me charts of physical exercises to do each day that would help my recovery.

Jane told me about Steve, a Craig patient in 2002 who had been a firefighter and smoke jumper for the Forest Service. He was part of a helicopter crew in Antarctica that was ferrying supplies and scientists when the helicopter crashed. Steve suffered spinal fractures that initially left him paralyzed from the waist down.

After his initial rehabilitation at Craig, Steve became Beverly and Jane's post-hospitalization therapy patient. As Steve's injuries healed, he was able to regain the ability to walk. After his therapy sessions concluded he contacted Jane outside of the clinic.

Jane, smiling broadly, said, "I suppose you would like to know if we still keep in touch?" Before I could answer she said, "We're engaged and will be married this September."

My connection with Craig's medical staff continued after my discharge and will probably continue for many years to come. I was able to be treated by Beverly and Jane as an outpatient (Chapter 13) and will be treated by many of Craig's other professionals during my future re-evaluation examinations.

8

Education: Lifelong Learning

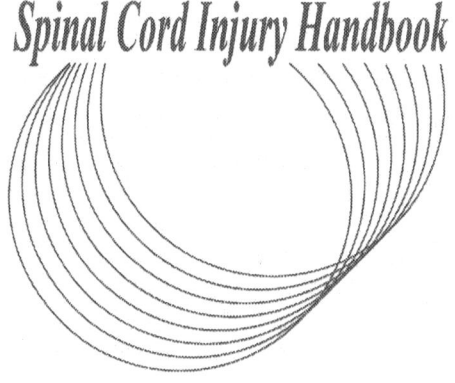

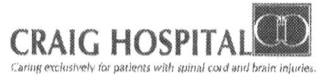

Fig. 8–1

Education, in its broadest meaning, begins when you enter Craig Hospital as a patient. Before I even saw my 3West room at Craig, I was already inundated with educational materials.

The Admissions Office is on the first floor of Craig's West building and the ambulance that brought me from Spalding Hospital parked right in front of Admissions. I hadn't even made it past Admissions when Jill, who was with me, was handed a small stack of orientation papers for me to read.

Later that day, or maybe the next morning (my first day or so at Craig being a blurred memory), Karen Mathias from Admissions, a great help in providing Jill with the information required to get me admitted to Craig, brought me the official admissions documents to sign. My legal background forced me to start to read the documents, evidently prepared by an attorney, but the small print and my powerlessness to change anything they said anyway, brought me back to reality. I simply stopped reading and signed the documents.

After Karen left, I read the orientation pamphlets and brochures stacked on the table next to my bed. There was Craig's *New Patient* booklet, smaller brochures on SCI and related brochures about various Craig departments. Still exhausted from the stress of transferring from Spalding, I really didn't absorb much of what I was reading. I didn't think about them again until after I moved to 3East.

The morning after my move, Patient and Family Education Coordinator Theresa (Terry) Chase paid me a visit. She gave me Craig's *Spinal Cord Injury Handbook*, a large three ring binder loaded with information about all aspects of SCI and told me her office was right across from my room. She'd be available any time I wanted to talk. After our brief conversation Terry turned—in her wheelchair—to go back to her office.

That was my first association with an amazing person who, in my opinion, is one of Craig's most valuable assets. I was awestruck when I watched her speed down the hallways, around corners and into rooms, utilizing her wheelchair as if it were a pair of power legs.

A Craig graduate, Terry arrived as a patient after being injured in an auto accident in 1988. Years later, immediately after becoming an RN and earning a Doctor of Nursing degree at the University of Colorado Health Science Center, she continued her teaching and education profession by filling Craig's newly formed position of Patient and Family Education Coordinator. When I met Terry she'd been at Craig nine years and had a reputation for being an educational godsend. (Before she came to her position, every department was responsible for planning and implementing its own classes.)

Terry not only coordinated patient and family education, but she also taught many class sessions, supported all patient educators and oversaw all educational materials, including: the resource library, textbooks, video tapes, brochures and handouts. She also arranged patient and family groups and outside speakers—many are Craig graduates who volunteered to share their stories with Craig patients and their families—for different departments in the hospital.

I considered Terry the resident troubleshooter, especially when the trouble was related in any way to education. In my case, she saved a man (me) from going through Internet withdrawal. When I needed help with the computers located in the education classroom, Terry took the time to show me exactly how to use each of the two computers and explained the limitations of the programs—basically they were "read only."

When I moved to 3East Terry made a point to remind me that my room, as well as all others on 3East, had high-speed and dial-up Internet connections. Unsure whether or not my old computer at home was compatible with Craig's connections, I asked Terry's advice. She didn't have an answer but made some phone calls to the Craig resident computer mavens and, within a day, came back with my answer. Of course, neither she nor I understood the technical parts of the answer but the plain part ("plug it in and use the dial-up") we understood.

Formal classroom education—required of all Craig patients when they are stable enough and their team physician approves—was conducted in a large room equipped with a big screen TV and VCR, a projector, two computers, charts and other teaching aids. The room, situated just off the public lounge area of 3East, was designed to accommodate students in wheelchairs or hospital beds as well as patients and visitors in regular chairs.

The classroom was conveniently located right across the floor from my room. By convenient I mean, if I didn't show up on time for a class (which rarely happened) it was very convenient for Terry to zoom across the hall to nab me.

Two to four one-hour classes were scheduled every week. All patients and their caregivers, families and visitors were welcome to attend most classes, the exception being the classes on sexuality where, for obvious reasons, they are limited to patients and their partners. Terry, being fully briefed on every new patient and on the medical progress of all others, was responsible for scheduling patients into the formal class rotations as soon as they are stable and cleared to attend by their team physician and therapists.

I started my classes on the eighth day of my Craig stay, my schedule indicating eighteen class sessions, the first ten were concerned with SCI, with an emphasis on healthy living after injury. Lecture topics included:

- An overview of SCI
- Bladder and bowel management
- Possible SCI complications
- Proper use of medications

- Nutrition
- Pain management
- Sexuality
- SCI research and more

While Terry or other Craig personnel taught most of the sessions, a number of sessions featured Craig grads or other SCI related speakers. The session I liked the most was the one that featured two employees of the Breckenridge Outdoor Education Center (BOEC)—one in a wheelchair—showing a video and equipment that enabled SCI and other handicapped people to ski or snowboard. The ease with which one instructor transferred from his wheelchair to the ski sled and back was inspiring.

My final eight formal class sessions came the week prior to my discharge and, along with Independent Living, described in a later chapter, were part of Craig's Re-Entry Program. The extremely important topics covered were:

- Loans, grants and other available financial resources
- Vocational rehabilitation
- Social skills
- Caregiver relationships
- Attendant care
- SCI research
- Sexuality

The format of the Re-Entry classes was different from the regular classes in that Re-Entry classes were not lectures but rather, group discussions. You stay with the same group for all the sessions and are encouraged to actively participate rather than only listen. The group leaders, depending on the topic being discussed, were doctors, Patient and Family Service counselors, psychologists or recreation therapists. In addition, one session leader is usually a peer counselor who once was an SCI patient who has since adapted and is living in the outside world as a "wheeler."

Education at Craig can be either formal or informal, structured or non-structured. Seminars and lectures held in the Education Room were formal and structured whereas certain peer lectures are somewhat structured but very informal. Of course, there is the undefined type of education you get just from observing what is going on around you.

Watching and talking with patients and former patients as their peer, was the best education imaginable for me. I didn't meet a single person at Craig who wasn't willing to discuss at length any topic relating to their SCI. There were frequent medical discussions, of course, but there was also hot debate over the best wheelchair makes and models that included about as much the same fervor as your average car debate.

Unfortunately for me, some of these discussions took place late at night in the lounge area right outside my door. As if that wasn't enough, sometimes JJ, a weeknight tech, joined the conversations and sent his laugh echoing up and down the halls. I was an extremely unappreciative audience.

Being open with and willing to talk about any subject I was conversant in, along with my age I suppose, made me the go-to patient for information and reinforcement. Having my own computer with Internet access also gave me a leg up on getting information. The fact that I sometimes took the role of teacher wasn't so bad, but one time it led to an interesting situation.

As part of the freshman curriculum at one of Colorado's top nursing schools, medical specialty rotations are required of each student. These rotations are designed to expose students to various nursing specialties such as emergency room, operating room, rehabilitative, pediatric and other nursing specialties. Swedish HealthONE Medical Center and Craig Hospital hosted a series of two-week rotations so that students could observe SCI patients one week and TBI patients the other. I happened to be at Craig when a group arrived for their two-week rotation.

One evening as I was mellowing out in my room after a grueling day of practicing standing up without help, the duty nurse and another nurse whom I had never met before, entered my room. The unfamiliar nurse introduced herself as supervisor of the visiting student nurses. She asked if I would agree to assist one of the students for an hour or so that evening as part of the SCI rotation training. Thinking they needed a "guinea pig" patient and never being one to turn down an opportunity to visit with a group of young would-be nurses, I quickly accepted without asking what I was needed for.

"I'll be back shortly," she said as she left my room, "You come highly recommended," she added as the door closed behind her.

"*Highly recommended for what?*"—I pondered. It didn't take long to find out, as there was a knock on my door within seconds.

"Come in," was followed by the supervisor entering and close behind, a beautiful, tall and confident looking nursing student. We were introduced and the supervisor, turning to leave, said to me, "She's all yours for the next two hours."

"What?" Taken totally by surprise, I conjured up images that made me wish I wasn't still paralyzed where it counted. *This is really cutting edge rehabilitation!* I kept my composure and invited my visitor to come into the living room area, sit on the couch and discuss the plans that I had no knowledge of.

The nursing student was extremely intelligent and well spoken. As it turned out, she informed me I was going to be her teacher, not a patient. Thinking I had been briefed beforehand, she burst into laughter when it dawned on her what I must have been thinking just a few moments earlier.

Because of my attitude, maturity and level of progress I had been chosen to have a student follow me through my entire routine of cathing, program and medications. I was expected to thoroughly explain the ins and outs of each step so that so she could learn, first-hand, the regular daily routine of an SCI patient.

I asked if she was squeamish or if she'd get upset observing the graphic procedures that were normal for me. She said that after spending her last rotation at Swedish observing many births, nothing would bother her. A few minutes later my Craig nurse came in and asked if she too could also observe my routine, how I managed to transfer from my wheelchair to the couch and back again, and how I set up the bathroom for taking a shower.

I was more than happy to show them and enjoyed explaining each step of my procedures to the student nurse. I answered her many questions as fully as I knew how. (I quietly thanked nurse Lilia Smith for teaching me so well.)

Before I could complete my evening routine, the nurse supervisor retrieved my student to take her to another room where there was an emergency going on with a quadriplegic respiratory problem. I never saw her again, but the next morning Craig nurse Debbie Shultz came to my room and relayed a message for me from my student. She wanted me to know that I was the best teacher she'd had in her rotations so far. Talk about a confidence builder!

Another educational opportunity occurred when I was a patient "Guinea Pig." A week or two after moving to 3East, I was trying to sleep, while at the same time dreading being aroused by the "leg measurers."

On this particular night, I was awakened and expected to see a measurer leaning over me with his/her tape. Instead, I saw what seemed to be the entire Mormon Tabernacle Choir standing around my bed. "Hi there," a woman in the group said, "Did we wake you?"

"No," I answered, "I never sleep well in a hospital."

The woman informed me that she was with student techs to learn the proper way to take leg measurements, then, without warning, she snapped on every room light, peeled back my bed covers and yanked up my long t-shirt (thank goodness I was wearing underwear.) She then proceeded to demonstrate each measurement position.

After her demonstration she invited each class member to try the procedure—on me, of course. After the sixth or seventh student had put freezing hands all over my legs, I had to protest. I needed sleep. The choir finally left, forgetting to turn off the lights and making me call the nurses' station for help.

Education doesn't just come from formal classes or on the job observations; education also comes from making mistakes. I learned this first hand when I became the victim of two different mistakes made by techs in training.

One evening shortly before my Foley Catheter was removed, I was in bed trying to fall asleep when my regular night tech, JJ, came into the room with three young women whom he introduced as techs in their first week of training. He said the women and their supervisor would be back at one o'clock to assist me in turning over. I said hello and went back to sleep.

Well, at one o'clock the techs returned and, keeping the room fairly dark and trying to be as quiet as possible, prepared to help me roll from my left side over to my right side. They split into two groups with one group standing on each side of my bed. Then, at the count of three, one group pushed me away from them while the other group pulled me towards them. I rolled over. Nicely done, but WHOOPS! Someone forgot about the Foley bag.

The proper procedure is to detach the bag from the side of my bed and, before turning me, swing it over me to the other side of the bed and attach it there. They didn't do that. The catheter tube was strapped to my thigh, so when the techs turned me, the tube tightened and squeezed the drainage bag through the bed rails. This opened the drain plug and dumped the bag's contents all over my feet and bed linens. Needless to say, this was a good learning experience for the student techs—who stayed and helped me clean up.

A week later, another tech had a learning experience in my room. Just after Kathy, my night shift nurse, left my room, my night tech came in to stock my supplies and check my linen supply. She checked my Foley bag and decided it needed emptying.

So after shutting the valve on the tube, she disconnected the bag, brought it into the bathroom, opened the drainage valve and let the contents empty into the toilet. She then re-attached the bag to the tube, hung it back on the bed, wished me a good night and left the room.

A few hours later my tech came back to turn me, bringing two "leg measurers" with her. Not sleeping soundly I was awakened by a strange liquid noise. "Squish, squish, squish," it went. I opened my eyes, and there in the dimly lit room I saw three people doing a dance on their tip-toes at the foot of my bed.

The tech had forgotten to close the drain valve on my Foley bag after she'd emptied it. So, with the drain wide open, the tube simply emptied me, for a few hours straight, through the bag and on to the floor. At least I stayed dry this time.

9

SCI: Accepting & Adapting

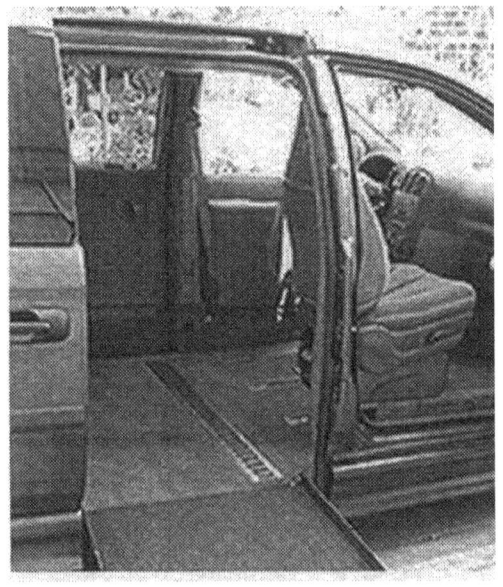

Fig. 9–1

One of the most difficult decisions to make is the one in which you force yourself to face the fact that your progress towards recovery may not advance any further. Sometimes, progress can be seen on a daily basis. Then, it seems unrealistic to consider that it will suddenly stop. But that may actually happen.

In my case, change was very slow in coming but rapid when it finally started. I reached a plateau though. The halt was barely noticeable at first but very noticeable later on.

My hardest time came when I had to accept that my injury was real and that, despite my bravado, I may be in the statistical majority and never fully recover. I was, and still am, convinced that my recovery will be close to complete but I don't know how long that will take.

Craig's treatment philosophy assumes patients will not recover past the stage that they are in at any given moment. This is the only philosophy to take as discharge plans must be made and necessary equipment and modifications selected and ordered. As a patient gets closer to discharge and/or if their needs require any changes, such as a different type of wheelchair or walker, liaison with insurance companies become ongoing and frequent. It is much easier to order equipment early based on prognosis and have it ready for patients to use (even if they don't end up needing it), than to hold off and having delays getting it fulfilled.

Craig Hospital provides for appropriate equipment through its wholly owned subsidiary, Adaptive Equipment Company (AEC). AEC specializes in durable medical equipment such as manual, power and computerized high-quad wheelchairs, bathroom equipment, ambulatory aids, hospital beds and assistive medical equipment. The company also maintains a loaner program and a seven-day a week emergency repair service to go along with AEC's seating and postural evaluation.

Being evaluated for a wheelchair and then having one fit to your requirements really awakens you to the reality of spinal cord injury (SCI). Accepting the probability of "permanent" injury is extremely difficult. It takes a lot of soul searching and introspection to finally reach the necessary acceptance. This acceptance is imperative because without it, you cannot put the required effort into your rehabilitation that will help you improve.

Speaking only for myself, my subconscious couldn't grasp the reality that I might not improve, even through hard work and medication, even though I believed that anything could happen if a person tried hard enough. I thought nothing of it when I received a manual wheelchair, but when OT Dana Lee and PT Hugh Simson told me that they were going to fit me for a power chair, (*A power chair,* I thought. *They're for seriously injured people, not someone like me!*) I realized how serious my injury was. I had to get down to the business of adapting to the situation—after all, I had been at Craig almost a month already.

Up until this point my association with Jaime Hoffman, my Patient & Family Service Counselor, was brief, pleasant and unproductive. I had no idea how important she was going to be to my rehabilitation, as I thought of her basically as the beautiful, well-dressed woman who kept bringing me things to read.

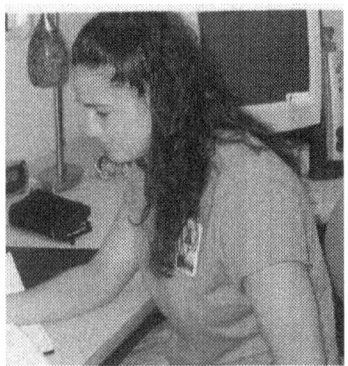

Jaime   Fig. 9–2

When I finally came to realize the possible ramifications the SCI may have on my life and living style, such as limited travel and mobility and no driving, I also realized how important Jaime was going to be to help me adapt to my condition and keep my lifestyle as close to normal as possible.

Her duties as a counselor were more far-reaching than I had first imagined. I also hadn't imagined the number of Family Service Counselors there were at Craig. To my surprise, Craig employed sixteen counselors including two directors (inpatient and outpatient), nine SCI counselors and five traumatic brain injury (TBI) counselors.

Not only did Jaime and the other counselors interact with patients, but they also were the direct link with insurance companies, landlords, local, state and federal agencies and facilitators of a smooth flow of an unbelievable volume of paperwork.

As a member of my rehabilitation team, Jaime was always bringing me forms to sign and applications to fill out. For instance, one of the packets she brought was a survey of all the rooms in my house. She'd use my survey to determine what modifications my townhouse would need and then get some companies to bid on the cost of modifications. One of the companies specialized in installing inside and outside elevators and lifts.

My first question to Jaime after I received this packet was "Why do I need this? My home won't need any modification."

"Herb," she started, "You live in a *three-story* house."

"Oh, Yeah."

I live in a three-story townhouse in Breckenridge, a small town situated close to the Continental Divide at an altitude of 9600 feet.

At my first and second team rehab conferences, the staff stated it was highly unlikely I would be able to return to Breckenridge upon discharge. I was the only person at the conference who was positive I would go home, despite recommendations to the contrary, and despite my daughter Jill's insistence that I stay at her home in nearby Lone Tree.

Jaime understood how serious I was about returning to Breckenridge and, by having me fill out the survey, she made me aware of the hardships I might encounter. For example, I had to ask myself how I planned to get groceries out of my car, conquer three flights of stairs and reach high pantry shelves if I was unable to walk.

As my rehabilitation progressed, Jaime would bring me different pamphlets and packets regarding Medicaid, state and local financial assistance programs, assistive equipment and more. She also kept in contact with my daughter and son-in-law to make sure their house was accessible for me and made sure that all aspects of my adapting to any environmental changes caused by my SCI were monitored and communicated to the appropriate people.

Part of adapting to the situation is re-learning how to do things that prior to SCI were taken for granted, like something as simple as taking a shower or as hard as parallel parking. After accepting the permanence of my new situation, this re-learning experience became a challenge and because of this, brought an element of fun to rehab. Not only did I enjoy the challenge, I enjoyed watching others succeeding in doing what I considered even greater challenges. (Nothing was more rewarding than seeing a quadriplegic patient feeding himself for the first time because he learned how to use his limited recovered muscle strength.)

As I noted in a previous chapter, my fellow patient Mark was known for his outgoing personality and affable nature. His recovery from paralysis to walking with forearm crutches was an inspiration to everyone and he made sure everyone was aware of his progress when he walked with the crutches around 3East, talking to patients and staff, and organizing activities.

One of Mark's rituals was to stop by a few rooms in the evening and say good night to their occupants. One of these occupants was Courtney Ferrall, a vivacious seventeen year old (*see Chapter 14 for her story*) and her mother, Millie, who was always with her. After many days of these visits Courtney, a joker herself, decided to play a trick on Mark.

One evening, with Millie's approval and help, Courtney waited for Mark to start his nightly rounds and then wheeled herself down to Mark's room. She then transferred from her wheelchair into Mark's bed, where she made herself comfortable, turned down the lights, turned on the TV and waited.

After a while, Mark opened the door, put down his crutches and, without looking, flopped down on his bed. Millie, who was hiding behind the door with her always-ready camera, stepped out and snapped a photograph just as Mark, surprised but laughing, realized he'd narrowly missed landing on the much smaller young woman in his bed—Courtney.

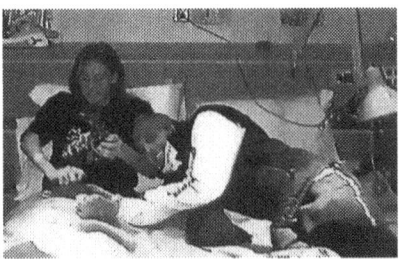

Mark Flopping on His Bed While Courtney Cringes Fig. 9–3

This type of playfulness goes a long way in helping SCI patients understand that an injury doesn't have to lessen their sense of humor. In fact, many patients used their ability of introspection to enhance their sense of humor and perhaps become even more childlike. For some patients this reversion to childhood only meant going back a few years, while for others it meant going back a few decades. (One of the more rewarding aspects of interacting with and observing other patients was witnessing their transition from sadness and depression to happiness and serenity.)

While taking inspiration from Mark and Courtney's antics, as well as from talking to and enjoying the feedback and interactions with many other patients, I worked as hard as I could with OT Dana and PT Hugh to make as much headway as possible. So far, Hugh had guided me through a series of challenges and exercises that aided my ability to regain some feeling and strength in my legs.

Hugh's challenges started with a machine that looked like something out of a Frankenstein movie. It allowed me to crank myself into a standing position while strapped in so I wouldn't fall. This progressed to using the parallel bars to pull myself up into a standing position. With this, I felt an even stronger urge to teach myself to walk again.

When Hugh first brought me to the parallel bars, I had to learn how to park my wheelchair and pull myself up while trying to push up with my weakened legs. At first, my great upper body strength was all I could rely on, but eventually I was able to push up with my legs. After standing up, Hugh had me try to walk a few steps while holding on to the bars. No go. I had no feeling in my legs and, despite a few clearly audible "C'mon legs," from me, my brain just could not get the message down to my legs to move.

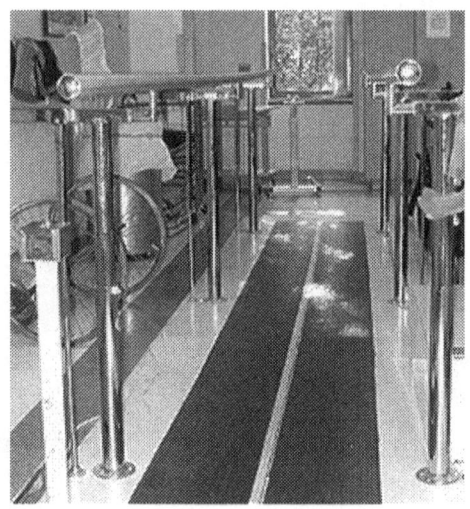

Parallel Bars   Fig. 9–4

As I was unable to walk by myself, Hugh had me concentrate on doing balancing exercises while standing in one spot. This, I could do fairly easily. Despite feeling no sensation whatsoever in my feet or butt, I learned to keep my balance by using visual references in the room and by judging where my feet were based on the feeling in my hips and thighs.

While Hugh was working on my leg strength with physical therapy, Dana was working on my domestic abilities with occupational therapy. Having already proven my superior skills in the area of kitchen clean up and room vacuuming, my next assignment was preparing a meal for myself.

Dana explained that she saw no problems with my ability to "eat" as she had observed me a few times at lunch, but she wanted to make sure that, when I was discharged from Craig, I could successfully plan, cook and enjoy a nutritious dinner all by myself. Sounded good to me.

Late one afternoon Dana came by my room and asked what my favorite dinner was. "Chicken," I replied, "Baked, fried, boiled or whatever."

"How does Chicken Parmesan with twice baked mashed potatoes and broccoli sound," she replied.

"Great. When do we eat?"

Dana said I could plan to have Chicken Parmesan for lunch in a couple of days but first I'd have to get the ingredients. I looked at her smile. Suckered again! I'd need a winter coat for the next morning's OT class because I would be wheeling a few blocks to Safeway to buy what was needed to make the chicken recipe. Another patient was in charge of preparing the potatoes and broccoli. We'd combine our efforts to present a meal for five.

The next morning I put on my ski jacket and gloves, met Dana at the elevator and off we went towards Safeway.—(Of course, I had no idea where Safeway was or what I was expected to do when I got there, but I would soon find out.) The entire excursion was planned to teach me how to maneuver my power wheelchair down sidewalks (keep it straight), across busy intersections (look both ways first), up small inclines (slow and steady) and through some muddy and/or snowy areas (don't stop in the middle).

When Dana and I arrived at Safeway, she handed me a shopping list and said, "Here's the list, go shopping."

I looked at the list and started to drive myself up the aisle to look for corn flake crumbs, cheese, chicken cutlets, eggs and cooking oil. I noticed that the cheese on the list was Mozzarella not Parmesan so I pointed it out to Dana.

"I don't care for Parmesan," Dana said. "I'll be eating lunch with you, go ahead and get Mozzarella instead."

That sounded OK to me so I drove around Safeway like a pro, luckily finding everything I needed on shelves I could reach. After going through the checkout without any problems we headed back to the 3West kitchen where, under Dana's watchful eye, I put the chicken in a marked storage bag then into the refrigerator and placed the other ingredients into the pantry.

The next morning I eagerly raced across the skybridge towards the 3West kitchen to prepare one of my favorite meals. Just as I rolled into the gym I met Dana on her way out. "Small problem," she said. "The girl making the side dishes needs another hour. She's using all the pans we need." My salivating stopped immediately but Dana just smiled and told me to, "Wait right there. I'll be back shortly."

I went into the gym, wheeled over to the kitchen and sat there enjoying the intense cheese and garlic aroma from the potatoes. Everything looked ready to go so I hoped Dana would be back with good news.

A few minutes later Dana returned and ordered me to grab the chicken and other ingredients and head for the 2West gym. (2West was the TBI floor.) I had never been there before but soon realized it was almost identical to 3West. Once there, I was ready to be put to the test.

The equipment on the second floor was not the same as on the third floor, but it didn't matter to me as long as I could reach everything from my wheelchair. The bowls and baking pans were easy to reach so I set about preparing the breading, dipping the filets and putting them into the pre-heated oven. Waiting for the chicken to bake gave me enough time to wash and dry the utensils I had just used and then wait for the chicken to be cooked enough to lay on the cheese. As I placed the Mozzarella strips on the sizzling chicken filets, I glanced up and saw that Dana, plus a few PTs from the TBI floor, was looking in the kitchen sniffing out the source of the aroma filling the gym.

After the chicken was done and covered with aluminum foil, I had to clean up the kitchen. (I pleaded unsuccessfully with Dana to try to get out of it.) We hurried back to the 3West gym where the other chef and her OT were waiting with the potatoes and broccoli. Dana informed me I had passed my "independent meal preparation test" with flying colors. My reward? A terrific lunch.

Right after my cooking adventure, I was back to serious work. Hugh had me walking on the mat between the parallel bars. I was awkward, had no balance and, due to a Sciatic nerve condition, was having back pain. In addition, although I had increased feeling down my legs, I still had no feeling below my ankles. This didn't deter Hugh from pushing me further and further.

I kept trying even though I felt weak and every so often a knee would buckle slightly and I would have to grab the bars for support. After a few hours of doing this, Hugh said that I was ready to try crutches. I disagreed. *I can't be ready. I don't have any balance or strength to support my weight.* .

Hugh, of course, was right, as I am sure he had seen this before. He went to an equipment locker and came back with two forearm crutches, identical except one was red and the other blue. I felt a little awkward standing there with the two different color crutches.

After demonstrating how to walk by using the opposite leg and crutch in rhythm, Hugh said I should give it a try. The left crutch was moved forward along with the right leg and then the right crutch was moved forward with the left leg. Hesitantly, I moved my left leg along with the right crutch, stopped, and then moved my right leg along with the left crutch. To my great surprise, I didn't trip myself or fall down!

For the next few PT sessions Hugh and I worked on me getting out of the wheelchair to a standing position, putting on the crutches and walking around the gym and the 3West hallways. At all times, I wore a chest belt that Hugh could grab on to in case I stumbled or otherwise lost my balance. There were a few instances when Hugh had to grab it but I never fell or even came close to falling.

This process was exhausting and caused a lot of back pain but I didn't stop. I had to progress. Luckily Hugh carried a water bottle for me, as I needed a thirst quencher constantly.

Many times during this hallway walking practice, I passed nurses, techs and other staff members. Without exception, each person, like Emily Jones of House-keeping, would offer "Great Job," or "Look at you go." These unsolicited cheers boosted my confidence and gave me the encouragement to pass by the Patient & Family Service office and give Jaime a "thumbs up" sign.

Once I almost bumped into Dr. Hsu as he rounded a corner. He stared at me then said, "Mr. Tabak, you are causing me to do a lot of extra paperwork. Every time I think you have reached maximum recovery, you fool me. Now I have to re-write your prognosis. Again." He laughed, and then went on his way.

I was practicing with my forearm crutches another time when I met Craig's President, Dennis O'Malley. I was literally stumbling down the hall on 1 West near the Craig Hospital Gift Shop when I stubbed the point of one of my crutches into the floor and nearly lost my balance. Struggling to stay on my feet, I inadvertently swung the other crutch into the air as Hugh grabbed my chest belt. As the crutch went up, it narrowly missed clipping a gentleman's head. The head belonged to Dennis O'Malley.

With a quick smile and a comment about how glad he was that I missed him, Dennis stopped and chatted with us for a few moments and then, wishing me continued success, turned and walked into his office.

Since I was getting closer to my discharge date but still not able to walk by myself or stop using a wheelchair for mobility, it was time to see if adaptation to most real-world environments had progressed to the point of self-sufficiency. I had read all the handouts from Jaime and Terry covering everything from traveling to bladder control but now Hugh and Dana were going to find out if I'd be able to apply the information.

One afternoon Hugh asked me if I was ready to go on outings outside the hospital, private outings with my visitors or even outings by myself, if I stayed close to the hospital. Dr. Hsu and my nurses had approved me, and so had he. If I felt comfortable going out, Hugh would help me make it happen. He'd approved me going out in either a manual or power wheelchair or a walker but not using just the forearm crutches.

I was ready. Hugh said that he would use the equipment in the transfer room to test me. He led me to the transfer room down in the basement of the West building. I'd never been there before and when he opened the door I wheeled myself into a room filled with the most amazing teaching aids I could ever imagine. Holding a Commercial Pilot's License, I had received many hours of flight training in airplane simulators but that did not prepare me for what was in the transfer room.

At first glance there appeared to be a full size black Honda automobile sitting to the left of the doorway. A closer look revealed the car actually started at the firewall and had no front end. Otherwise, it was a standard Honda with a complete interior, trunk, tires and trim.

Next, I saw a set of about six rows of complete commercial airliner seats, with an aisle dividing three seats on one side from two on the other side. Then, I noticed a double bed, a toilet, commode seats, shower benches and equipment I didn't even recognize. Hugh laughed when he saw the look on my face, and then said, "Let's start with the car so you can go out with Jill and Michael."

Within a few minutes I learned how to transfer with ease from the wheelchair into the Honda seat. Naturally, in the real world, someone would have to fold up my wheelchair and put it into the car trunk, but at this time, that wasn't my problem.

At a later session I learned how to navigate up the aisle of an airplane and Dana gave me a session on getting on and off the bed. I was already proficient at using the bathroom and shower equipment so I didn't spend any time on them. But still, there was one transfer I could never quite master.

I could not transfer from my wheelchair or commode chair to my hospital bed. The first week or so I had no trouble doing this but then I had trouble that lasted until I received a normal double bed. The reason for this difficulty was an example of compromise where you give up something in return for receiving something else. In my case, I gave up ease of transfer for being comfortable in bed.

I found I couldn't sit up in bed to read or watch TV without sliding down the sheets. To alleviate this problem, a large foam rubber mattress cover was installed on my bed. Even though it was placed under the bed sheets, it would prevent me from sliding down the bed when I was trying to sit up.

However, with one problem solved, another one was created—transferring into bed. The mattress cover was so bulky that it raised the height of the bed about 3 inches. This made the transfer board higher on the bed and lower on the wheelchair or commode chair. Transferring from the bed to either chair was easy as I just slid downhill into the chair. Getting back into bed was another matter.

Transferring from the wheelchair to the bed was slightly easier than from the commode chair to the bed, especially if I was wearing sweat pants. I simply placed one end of the board on the bed, placed the other end under my thigh in the wheelchair, grabbed onto the bed's side rails with both hands and pulled myself up the board and onto the bed.

The real problem arose when transferring from the commode chair. This chair was used for my program or taking a shower so when I was ready to get into bed I usually had a bare bottom or was wearing underwear. Since I couldn't slide uphill on the board in this condition—not if I wanted any skin left on my thighs—, I had to transfer from the seat to the bed by placing my hands on the bed or chair arm, pushing down with my arms, swinging my butt over a few inches and sitting down on the board, hopefully a few inches further up the board. Knowing I wouldn't slide down the board if it had contact with my skin, I repeated this maneuver a few more times as I inched my way up the board and into bed.

After mastering indoor mobility I decided to put my newly found freedom to the test. This test arrived a few days later when Olivia, my friend from Florida, came to visit. Feeling my oats and wanting to enjoy the outdoors, I suggested we walk to the *All For the Better Gourmet Ice Cream Shop* at the corner of Hampden and Clarkson, about a block from the hospital.

Olivia agreed, so I cranked up my walker and signed out at the nurses' station. We took the elevator to the first floor and, with me trying to keep a steady but not fast pace, left the building. Walking downhill towards the corner, I took it slowly and carefully, and had a reasonably easy time easing down the extremely steep hill to the ice cream shop.

Once at the shop Olivia and I ordered some absolutely delicious ice cream and sat down to enjoy it although the chairs felt like cement slabs even to someone who has no feeling in his butt.

The jaunt back to Craig wasn't so easy. I found myself struggling to walk uphill and the grade was so steep I almost had to carry my walker. Olivia was getting nervous, thinking I might fall, but I assured her my balance and strength were fine and if I just walked slowly I could make it.

At one point I stopped to catch my breath and Olivia offered to go back to 3East and have a tech bring my power chair. (I was thinking a gurney would be better.) But, I refused her offer and struggled to continue. I eventually made it back to the entrance and back up to my room. I collapsed on my couch and wished I'd been in better shape. (And had saved some of the ice cream!)

10

The Rehab Puzzle:
Making The Pieces Fit

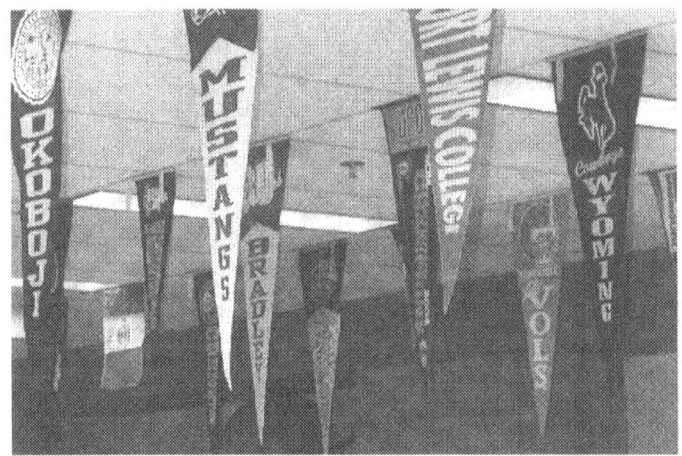

Fig. 10–1

After my first four weeks of rehabilitation, the pieces of the rehab puzzle started to come into focus and fit together. Education classes that had been interesting but outside my realm of understanding, suddenly clicked with me. I finally correlated the education information with the procedures in PT and OT classes. It was putting theory into practice. Here's an example.

When I first got to Craig I was constantly reminded to shift my weight in the seat of my wheelchair. I knew one reason for shifting was to aid circulation in the lower extremities. But, while attending one of my first SCI education classes, I learned there are other reasons for it too. The main one is to avoid getting body sores.

Checking my skin for redness or other abnormalities that could indicate possible areas of rubbing became a daily routine. I was given a mirror attached to a long, flexible rod (Fig.10–2) and taught how to use it while lying in bed. By bending the rod I could change the angle of the mirror to inspect every part of my body I had never seen before (and hope never to see again).

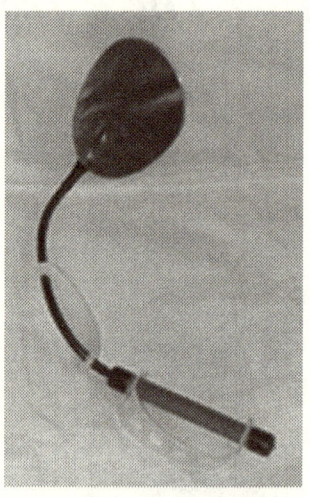

Mirror   Fig. 10–2

Body sores, also known as skin sores, pressure sores or bed sores, are caused by lying in bed in one position too long, or by sitting in a wheelchair in the same position too long. They're a common occurrence for people who have no sensory perception or who are paralyzed and cannot move. The danger that comes from getting a sore, is that it can get infected, which may not only be painful, but may lead to possibly fatal complications. Christopher Reeve, despite his remarkable progress to overcome his SCI, succumbed to cardiac arrest caused by a pressure sore systemic infection.

I was extremely negligent doing regular weight shifts in both my manual and power wheelchairs. Outside of class, a nurse or PT would have to remind me to do a weight shift but in class, it was easy to remember. There was always one or two quadriplegics who had a built in timer in their large power chairs. They would set the timer to ring at prescribed times between weight shifts and then when it went off, they activated their chairs to tilt them to the desired angle and thus, create a weight shift. I simply picked one patient and each time that patient's timer rang, I locked my chair brakes, lifted myself up out of the chair seat with my arms, and stayed in that position for thirty seconds while I gave my bottom a break.

Another way to reduce the possibility of getting body sores, and also to protect your feet and toes from injury, is to wear loose fitting clothing and footwear. When I first heard about this it did not make sense to me. My experience was that loose fitting clothing bunched up and caused wedgies, more irritation, not less. The techs assured me I was wrong. My PT insisted on loose fitting foot protection.

I finally gave in and said I would try it their way. I asked Jill to purchase an extra *extra* large (XXL) sweat suit for me. I also asked her for a pair of inexpensive sneakers size 11 ½ or 12, at least a full size larger than my normal 10. Wearing the sweat suit and huge shoes made me look like a baggy-pants clown. I had to admit they were comfortable to exercise or wheel around my wheelchair in.

Later in my rehabilitation, I found it necessary to tape my sweat pants tight at the ankles to prevent stepping on them when I was walking with the walker or crutches or doing exercises on the gym mats.

With almost every phase of my rehabilitation program showing improvement, at that time, I was, and still am, disappointed that I haven't had full improvement in my bowel function program, commonly just called *The Program*.

One of the major ramifications of a T-10 and below SCI is paralysis of the bladder and part of the large intestine. Not only is there loss of sensory ability, but also of motor function. This translates into losing your ability into voluntarily urinate or move your bowels as well as losing the feeling of needing to.

The bladder must be emptied to prevent muscle damage from overextension, Urinary Tract Infection (UTI) or kidney damage. This is easily taken care of by using a Foley Catheter at first, and then switching to some form of Intermittent Catheterization (IC). While the muscles controlling the bladder may not recover for a long time, if ever, proper catheterization techniques will help you in regaining sensation and the urge to urinate.

Elimination of digestive process waste is essential to maintaining a healthy body and is especially critical to a person with a SCI. For many people with spinal cord injuries the ability for the nerves to send the proper signal to the brain regarding the sensation to have a bowel movement, or even the ability to control the movement, is lost. Because of this bowel management is not easy, and requires discipline to accomplish.

The human body, however, is an interesting machine. It knows waste elimination is essential and, if properly trained, its muscles can assist in causing this function to occur. This requires that the affected person must establish and maintain a complete bowel program consisting of proper diet and medications, proper fluid intake, regular physical activity and a schedule.

Proper diet and food intake assist the body in getting the required nutrients. Keeping yourself up to date on your medications' side effects can minimize adverse reactions that are counterproductive to a proper bowel movement. Regular physical activity (anything from getting out of bed, walking or participating in any sport) also helps stimulate proper bowel function.

The most important part of the bowel program is sticking to a consistent schedule. Because the body will adjust to that schedule, it is essential that the bowel program be done at the exact same time every day. When this is accomplished, taking care of this essential function becomes routine.

Once I understood the goals attached to most rehabilitation procedures and compared them to my own specific goals, more pieces of what seemed to be a giant puzzle came together. The puzzle pieces included schedules, meal times, computer access, mandatory classes, weekend gym use, ability (and written permission) to move about my room and around 3East, access to the large medical video library and almost everything else that was a regular part of Craig.

Scheduled formal PT and OT classes, both individual and group, were held Monday through Friday from as early as eight o'clock in the morning to four o'clock in the afternoon. There were no classes on weekends so the 3West gym was usually dark and quiet. However, there were some die-hards like myself who wanted to use the gym on weekends when we weren't seeing visitors.

At the beginning of my rehab at Craig, the only non-supervised gym programs that my physical therapist, Hugh, approved me for were using the small pulley weights and doing exercises on the mats. As I progressed, he encouraged me to use the parallel bars for balance and walking exercises. Many times on a Saturday or Sunday, especially when the weather was too cold to go outside, I wheeled over to the gym. The pool was not open and supervised on the weekend. Too bad, I would have luxuriated in its warm water after a week of strenuous therapy.

Another patient who would have liked weekend access to the pool was Drew Wills, an attorney from Colorado Springs who lived a few rooms down from me. Drew and his wife, Jeanie, always seemed to spend a lot of time in the pool, but it just so happened Drew was scheduled for the session right before mine on most days.

Jeanie completely took to heart Craig's philosophy of family participation in a patient's rehab and tried to join Drew in the pool whenever she could. It became my routine to look for them, and most of the time, when my pool therapy didn't require use of the entire pool, I was happy to share my session with them. (*Drew's story can be found in Chapter 14*)

Sometimes the pool became the "Ole Watering Hole" as it seemed that everyone from 3East showed up at the same time for one reason or another. One time I was just being lifted out of the water when Courtney, Drew and two other 3East patients showed up at the same time. Drew had the next scheduled session, followed by Courtney but everyone else just dropped in. This must have driven Carol, the pool PT, nuts because not only did she have her patients crowding around the pool in wheelchairs, but she also got their family members, including Courtney's mother Millie and Drew's wife Jeanie, sitting in the guest chairs.

The actual pool therapy sessions were difficult but, as a part of the rehab puzzle, they were easy to understand. It surprised me when I found out for myself that I could do things with my body while in water that I couldn't even think of doing out of the water. From the very start of my pool therapy I was able to stand in the pool when I couldn't even pull myself into a standing position outside the pool. It's a weightless phenomenon that, for some reason, is even stronger in warm water.

PT pool sessions were designed to give patients maximum results from exercising the muscles that are not exercised in the gym, namely legs.

As my physical strength improved and as I gained more mobility working with Hugh, Carol increased the size of my leg weights in the pool and assigned more advanced exercises for me to do. Now, I not only had to walk across the pool without assistance, but I also had to walk a black line painted on the bottom of the pool. (Trying to keep my balance, I could relate to what figure skaters go through to balance on one skate.)

Another exercise was walking across the pool while balancing on a square pipe that Carol, or Carol's volunteer Amanda had dropped into the pool. These exercises were challenging and fun at the same time. I always had a feeling of accomplishment when I completed them.

Carol and Hugh kept each other appraised of my progress, so there was no chance of my slacking off in either therapist's class. When Carol found out that I had progressed from wheelchair to walker, even if just for short periods of time, she stopped using the lift to get me into the pool. *Thanks Hugh.* Instead, I had to wheel to the edge of the pool steps, pull myself out of the chair by using the pool's handrails and then let Carol assist me as I worked my way down the seven steps one plod at a time.

Getting out of the pool was the same procedure, only in reverse. I didn't need Carol's assistance in going up the steps because I was developing more strength in my legs. When I reached the top step, Amanda or another pool volunteer hosed me down and then brought my wheelchair over. Still holding on to the railing with one hand, I was able to turn around and lower myself into the chair. Near the end of my stay at Craig my mobility had improved to the point where I could traverse the pool stairs in both directions without any assistance.

The central piece of the puzzle snapped together with the others when my PT and OT sessions merged. When Hugh came to the conclusion that, with proper guidance (translate: extreme bullying), I would definitely be able to walk on my own, he met with OTs Donna and Dana and they all agreed that although they knew how painful it was going to be for me, PT and OT sessions would from then on concentrate on walking practice.

My sciatic nerve condition still flared up in my right hip and leg if I stood up for any length of time. To make matters worse, my Parkinson's would decide to rear its unwanted head to make it hard to move my feet. I must have looked like a real clod trying to walk down the halls on the days when everything was flaring up. Luckily, most days, only one or two things bothered me, and that only was after an hour or so of walking.

The hardest exercise for me was learning to ascend and descend stairs using the forearm crutches. Whether going up the stairs or down, you remove the crutch from the arm next to the railing and hold it horizontal to the ground with the other hand while maintaining a grip with the same hand on the remaining crutch's handle.

Going up the stairs was a breeze for me as my leg muscles had regained a lot of strength. Actually, I was able to get up the stairs without using the crutches at all.

Going down the stairs was another story. For some physiological reason, my knees could not hold my body weight without buckling, so I was forced to use both forearm crutches. Holding the crutches the same way as before, you put the crutch down first on the step you are going to and then the leg on the same side as the crutch followed by the rail-side leg.

I practiced this for hours—on what seemed to be every stairwell in Craig—combined with just walking the Craig hallways. My daily OT classes just continued with this practice after my daily PT classes were over.

Believe it or not, just walking the hallways was actually the most difficult exercise of all, especially when using the forearm crutches. Using the walker was relatively simple as all I had to do was stand up, lean forward and place both hands on the walker bar and move my legs. It was a little awkward at first but once I got a rhythm going it became smoother and easier.

Walking with the forearm crutches was the antithesis of ease. First off, the crutches are physically uncomfortable, and if they are not properly adjusted for your height, using them can be either painful or dangerous. The bottom part of the crutch leg could be raised or lowered easily so all I did was put my arms into the forearm brace, clench my hands around the handles and stand there while Hugh adjusted the legs.

Secondly, in order to maintain proper balance and not fall, I had to coordinate moving the crutch with moving the opposite leg. Sounds easy, doesn't it? It was just like taking dancing lessons and hearing the instructor repeating, "One, two, three—One, two, three…" except my legs wouldn't stay with the beat. It's like telling people to swing their arms while walking. They do it just fine when they're not thinking about it, but think about it and their arms and legs try to move in tandem.

Most days walking went well and, if I kept in sync, I had no trouble. Those days I had plenty of stamina and enjoyed walking all over the hospital. Some other days were disasters. I just couldn't coordinate my legs and, worst of all, I had little stamina. It was all I could do to walk out of the gym and around one corridor without having to sit and rest. C'est la vie!

The scariest exercise was walking outdoors in snow and ice while using forearm crutches, a feat I compared to walking on stilts across the tundra. A few times Hugh and Dana dragged me out into the Colorado winter right after a new snowfall had left a few more inches of the white stuff on the ground.

Each snow slalom session was short and right to the point. I walked down a long ramp, up and down two curbs, across the parking lot and back inside. The ramp usually had little snow on it because it had been cleared. The curbs, on the other hand, had deep packed snow on top of ice on them and the parking lot had a combination of snow, ice and slush. Luckily for me the low temperatures bothered Dana so sessions with her were short. I didn't want her to be uncomfortable after all. On the other hand, Hugh is a New Brunswick raised Canadian who spent quite a bit of time in the Calgary area and just thrived in cold weather. Damn it anyhow!

Less than two weeks before my discharge, PT Hugh left Craig to pursue another career opportunity. After he left, I thought I would get a reprieve for my few remaining days, but no such luck. Picking up right where Hugh left off was PT Tam Chamberlain. Tam didn't let me miss one step as she deftly assumed command of my therapy. Of course, this was just a natural thing for Tam who had been a PT at Craig for seven years and before that, she served eight years active duty with the U.S. Army, attaining the rank of Captain. She was a helicopter pilot, including being a maintenance test pilot on Blackhawk Helicopters. In actuality, she was the perfect addition to my rehab to help me transition from being paraplegic to being ambulatory.

As more and more puzzle pieces fit together I found that my days seemed to go by faster than before. I was in a groove and felt very comfortable with the daily routine especially when my rehab was going so well that even I could see the daily changes.

Each separate phase of rehab such as PT, OT, education, medication, physical strength and attitude had all reached the same level and were now working jointly rather than as distinct phases. The puzzle was complete.

11

Craig Research: Promising Possibilities

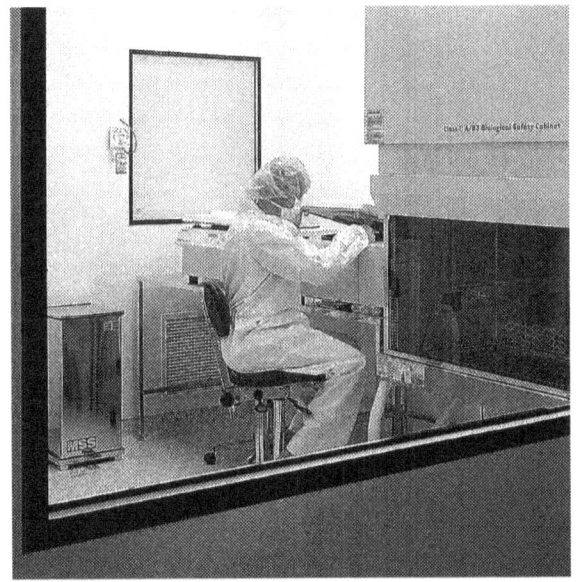

Fig. 11–1

I would be remiss if I didn't include at least a short chapter in *No Whining* about the research being done at Craig Hospital to find new treatments for patients with spinal cord injuries and traumatic brain injuries. Craig is a leader, in an innovative way, in the areas of SCI and TBI research.

Many well-known hospitals combine research facilities with clinical trial facilities, which was always the way it had been done in the past. Large universities, usually those with a medical school, became recipients of government and private research grants to study various medically related subjects.

Craig Hospital has a unique rehabilitation philosophy that maintains admission criteria covering only two areas, SCI and TBI. Because all patients are carefully screened and must meet these admission criteria, Craig has available one of the best patient research pools imaginable. Soon after being admitted to Craig, patients are asked for written permission to use their statistical records, (without identity disclosure, of course) for accumulating data to be used in the future.

My introduction to Craig's Research Department came the day Susie Charlifue came to my room on 3East to request I sign a consent form. At the time I had no real knowledge of what kind of research, if any, was done at Craig, or what research was planned for the future. She explained in detail what the consent form entailed and that the consent was for data collection only. I, and my medical information would remain anonymous.

After agreeing to sign the consent form, I asked Susie to fill me in on research at Craig. She briefly told me about some of the projects that had been done in the past and touched on a few of the current ones. I was surprised to find out that Craig has been active in research for many years.

Craig Hospital, a designated Model Systems Center, has been conducting SCI research for many years as part of its commitment to the treatment of SCI. Since 1974, Craig, in collaboration with Swedish HealthONE Medical Center and St. Anthony Central Hospital, has been the federally designated Rocky Mountain Regional Spinal Injury System (RMRSIS) and has been funded by the US Department of Education's National Institute on Disability and Rehabilitation Research (NIDRR). At the present time, Craig Hospital is one of the largest designated regional SCI centers and contributes more cases to the national SCI database than any other facility.

In addition to the research being done by the RMRSIS, Craig Hospital, since 1998, has also actively engaged in research as one of sixteen facilities that comprise the TBI Model Systems Program.

Historically, Craig Hospital is best known for its research in three areas: The clinical care of people with high level tetraplegia; the process of aging with spinal cord injury; and the development of outcome measures to document the degree in which people with disabilities return to active productive lifestyles.

One benefit of the Model System program is the environment created at Craig, which has given rise to the ability to obtain funding for additional research from other sources. Currently Craig Hospital is engaged in the following named research projects:

Spinal Cord Injury

A. Rocky Mountain Regional Spinal Injury System (NIDRR)

- Shoulder pain
- Spinal cord untethering and expansion duraplasty
- Recovery from pressure sore surgery
- Perimenopause in women with SCI
- Partners of men with SCI: Issues related to providing assistance
- Environmental barriers

B. Refining the Understanding of Aging with SCI (NIDRR)

- Secondary conditions from 5–25 years post-injury
- New analytic techniques with longitudinal datasets
- Chronic pain
- Access to and satisfaction with health services
- Personal assistance
- Spirituality and the effects on health outcomes, quality of life and well-being
- Perceived stress and self-reported problems
- Trends in quality of life and health

C. Fampridine-SR Clinical Trial (Acorda Therapeutics)

- Open-Label Extension to Evaluate Use of Oral Fampridine-SR in Subjects with Chronic, Incomplete SCI

D. Procord Clinical Trial (Proneuron Biotechnologies, Inc., Israel)

- A Phase II Multicenter, Randomized Study of Autologous Incubated Macrophages for Treatment of Complete SCI

E. Stem Cell Research (The Karolinska Institute, Sweden)

- A Joint Laboratory Study with the Karolinska Staff Involving Potential Human Stem Cell Therapies

F. Genetics and SCI Recovery

- Genes Influencing Recovery After SCI

G. Pfizer Pain Study (Pfizer Pharmaceuticals)

- Validation of Pain Measures

Traumatic Brain Injury

A. The Rocky Mountain Brain Injury System (NIDRR)

- Modanafil for Fatigue after TBI
- Social Communication Skills Training after TBI
- Outcomes and Environmental Factors after TBI

B. Mortality After TBI Rehabilitation (NIDRR)

- Life Expectancy and Cause of Death

(Click on www.craighospital.org/research for further information)

Thanks to the years of funding from the SCI Model Systems Program, Craig Hospital has been able to design and test many of the components which now constitute critical elements of the current treatment regime including the rehabilitation engineering program, the driver's training program, the community re-entry program and aspects of the vocational rehabilitation program.

Craig, through supporting its partners, receives immediate benefits in the form of "first use" of new procedures or techniques developed by the partner during research. A good example of how well this type of partnership can work is illustrated by the partnering between Craig Hospital and the Karolinska Institute of Stockholm, Sweden for the purpose of stem cell research.

The Karolinska Institute is home to the Nobel Prize and also maintains varied scientific research facilities that employ the services of approximately 2,000 MDs and PhDs. The Institute's long-term interest in SCI and collaboration with Craig has resulted in advancing the necessary knowledge towards achieving greater understanding of the answers obtained in animal research and their applications to human spinal cord injury treatment. Neurosurgeon Dr. Scott Falci of Craig Hospital is working with the Karolinska Institute on a project where human embryonic spinal cord tissue is used to attempt to restore function in laboratory animals.

To oversimplify the subject and to explain: Stem cells are neutral body cells that have not yet formed a specific identity of their own, e.g. skin cells, organ cells, heart muscle cells, etc. The most exciting trait of these cells is their ability to find their way to an injured area of the body and then morph into the specific cells needed to repair the injury. The research into this phenomenon is ongoing but still early and, while some reported cases of its use in animals is encouraging, there have been few human trials reported.

The possibilities stem cell research may open up are as astounding to us today as was the possibility of a cure for Polio must have been in our parents' day. If, and that's a big if, the regenerative traits of stem cells can be understood or even reproduced in a laboratory setting and successfully implanted into injured or ill people the regenerative traits of the cells could be used to heal spinal cord damage, reverse paralysis, regenerate brain cells and reverse the effects of TBI as well as be used to effect major recoveries in neurological and other areas.

Stem cell research, especially *embryonic* stem cell research, has become a political football being kicked around by politicians, some of whom have never taken the time to research the facts of this vital topic.

It is my opinion that the political and moral issues should be debated outside the medical arena so as to not interfere with the progress research is pointing to. An example of such progress was reported in the September 19, 2005 issue of *Proceedings of the National Academy of Sciences*. Researchers at the University of California, Irvine reported that injections of human stem cells into mice seemed to repair some of the damage caused by spinal cord injury.

In addition to the research listed previously, Craig Hospital recently received research grants for two other areas of study: The Efficacy of Massage Therapy (National Institute of Health) and The Impact of TBI on Female Endocrine Functioning (Colorado Traumatic Brain Injury Trust Fund). Dr. David Ripley MD is heading the research on Female Endocrine Functioning as the principal investigator. The research commenced July 1, 2005.

As I became stronger and able to maneuver my wheelchair around Craig Hospital grounds, I was always on the lookout for an ominous looking building that, in my mind, would probably look like an old chemistry lab. There, all this mysterious "Research" was taking place.

It wasn't until Medical Director Dr. Daniel Lammertse gave a lecture about research at Craig did I realize that Craig was actually a research partner not an entire research entity. This makes a lot of sense and benefits all concerned—by providing the patients for approved clinical trials, Craig saves its research partner much time, money and problems inherent with establishing their own patient sites.

The research being conducted at Craig Hospital is extremely important to the future treatment of SCI and TBI. Who knows what breakthroughs may happen right there, or if, in some small way, the research data collected on my injury and rehabilitation assists in a SCI treatment discovery. I'd like that.

12

Final Test: Independent Living

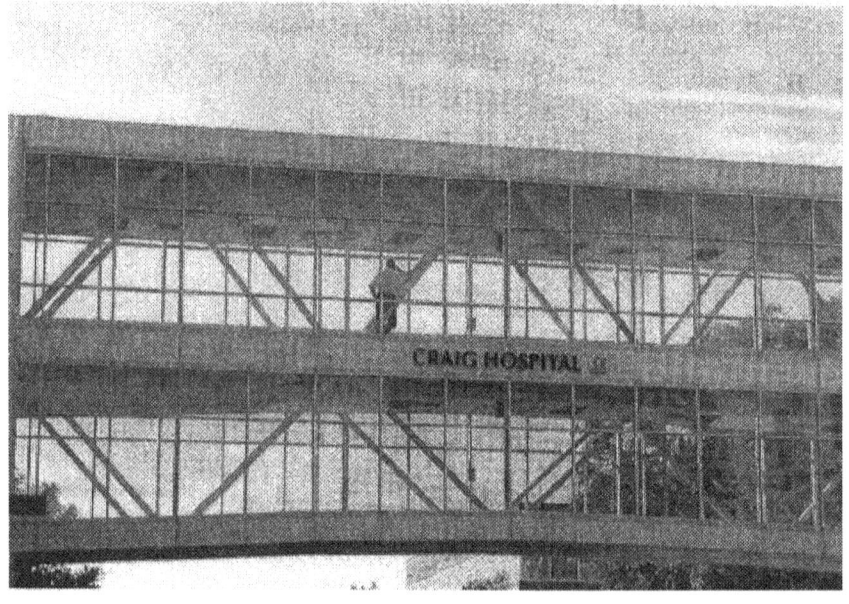

Fig. 12–1

About ten days before my expected date of discharge, my day nurse Peggy, informed me Dr. Hsu had approved placing me on Independent Living status for the remainder of my time at Craig. "It sounds impressive," I said, "but what exactly does it mean?"

Peggy replied, "It means that for your last few days here, you'll be completely on your own. You'll have to dress, shave, eat and do anything and everything else that has to be done without outside assistance. This means no help from me, the other nurses, techs or staff members." We'll still dispense your meds but you're going to have to go ask for them at the nurses' station."

Since I felt I had been fairly independent for a while already, this change in status didn't bother me one iota. After all, I was beginning to feel like an old timer at the place. As usual I was prematurely confident.

The next morning as I was getting ready to go to my scheduled PT session, two men from Housekeeping arrived toting parts of a double bed on a large hand truck. They came into my room and one of them asked, "Are you Herb?"

I nodded, he then explained that they were here to take my hospital bed and leave a standard double size bed.

"Wait just a doggone minute," I thought to myself, "How am I going to sit up in bed to watch TV or answer the phone?"

The two quickly detached all the cords from my hospital bed and wheeled it out to the hallway, hauled in the double bed parts and easily assembled them. After dropping the mattress on the frame, they wished me luck and disappeared down the hall, my old bed's wheels squeaking a medley of tunes as they went along.

Ginny, my day tech arrived a short while later with clean sheets and lots of new pillows, as she was aware that I would need major propping up in this new bed. I had only just adjusted to my hospital bed and was not looking forward to re-adjusting. My apprehension was warranted.

After a night or two trying to sleep, I asked Ginny to please rustle up either a stiffer mattress or a board I could put under the mattress. Unable to find a solution, Ginny forwarded my request to Housekeeping to see what they could do.

The very next morning, Housekeeping Supervisor Frank Ramirez came into my room, measured my bed, and left with a wave.

Late that afternoon two Maintenance Department employees brought a large piece of plywood to my room and placed it under my mattress. Sleeping problem solved!

With the sleeping problem taken care of, I phoned Jill and luckily found her still at home, but getting ready to leave to come to Craig. I told her about my new Independent Living status and asked her to stop at a supermarket on her way and pick up some microwave food as it looked like I was going to have the option of becoming my own cook or wheeling to the cafeteria for meals. Room Service was about to be canceled.

These were really just small adjustments to have to make to achieve full Independent Living status. Major changes, although unofficial, had already been made weeks before. Hugh had already "signed me off" after I was able to stand by myself and transfer easily from the wheelchair to the couch, bed, commode seat and shower bench. This permission to act on my own was the beginning of living as an independent, self-sufficient adult. Being able to shower by myself, do my evening bowel program alone and get in and out of bed unaided took the concepts of confidence and morale boosting to a new level.

The transition from total dependence to independence was slow in coming and just as subtle in occurring. A few times during my last week at Craig I sat on my couch just before getting into bed for the night, and tried to put into perspective the fact that only a few weeks previously I was totally reliant on others to attend to every aspect of my life. This was very difficult to comprehend and, even more difficult than comprehending, was stifling the fear that I'd regress. So far, so good!

Another thing that helped create an independent feeling in me was having my home computer at Craig so I could keep up with some of my consulting work and personal affairs.

One weekend in January, Jill and Michael retrieved my CPU and printer from Breckenridge and brought them, along with a present, to Craig. What was the present? A new flat screen monitor! It only took me about twenty minutes to wire the components, plug in the dial-up connection and to be on line and in business. I am convinced that the ability to spend a few hours a day doing my normal business routine as well as surfing the net late at night when I couldn't sleep—just as I did at home—helped speed up my rehabilitation just as much as the intense PT and OT did.

There is no way to truly measure how rehabilitation is positively impacted by the elimination of mental stress and anxiety, but in my situation, having the computer at hand and being able to take care of my personal affairs and business matters made a huge difference.

Other patients brought a sense of normalcy to their lives at Craig in various ways. Some did this by using laptops, some by decorating their rooms with school banners and pennants, some by having their Teddy Bear collection on their beds and some by surrounding themselves with family and friends. (*Family and friends is a subject I touch on in Chapter 15*).

Independent Living status can cause some unusual changes in your previous daily routine too. During the week, I usually woke up to Ginny knocking on my door and bringing me the day's breakfast menu. Now, I had to get myself awake and out of bed and then "supposedly" go to the 3West gym for breakfast. This change was not acceptable to me, not because I didn't want to eat with other patients, but because I wanted to use that time to be on my computer. Ginny understood, yet even though I was willing to miss eating breakfast, she was unable to let me starve. She somehow delivered a small breakfast tray to me every morning.

Supper was altogether different as there was a conflict between socializing in the gym and cooking in my room using the microwave oven. I think I managed to overcome this conflict by combining the two activities. Jill would bring me some of her family's leftovers so I could heat them up and have a great meal. But before heating them up, I would wheel over to the gym and pick up plates, utensils, napkins, salad, fruit and/or other desserts with trimmings and gain some socialization time in the process.

Living alone without the daily supervision that had been SOP for the previous seven weeks, left me feeling slightly abandoned. The severance would have been total except for the fact that it was considered too risky to allow patients to help themselves to their medications from the pharmacy. I now had to track down the nurse to get my meds at the appropriate time.

Being permitted to get out of bed without supervision or assistance meant I could get up in the middle of the night to sit on the living room couch, watch TV, play on the computer or do anything else I wanted. It was at these times temptation reared its ugly head. I don't know about other patients, but sometimes in the middle of the night I'd get food cravings that were hard to explain or even diffuse.

At Craig, I tried to keep the refrigerator reasonably well stocked with healthy snacks like fresh fruit, applesauce for taking pills, Gatorade or Caffeine Free Diet Pepsi, and any other edible odds or ends. But what I really wanted was chocolate, and I had lots of it.

Why is it when people visit hospital patients they follow some law that mandates they bring either flowers or candy? Flowers make me sneeze and after a few weeks at Craig, I had amassed at least ten boxes of chocolates of all brands, types, shapes, fillings and sizes. I tried giving the chocolates away to other patients but they had the same problem, so they wouldn't take them. A couple of nurses took two boxes off my hands and some techs dropped in now and then and ate a few of the morsels but they refused to take a box with them.

After a while I realized that if I continued to eat chocolate in the middle of the night I was going to get very sick and might have to stay past my discharge date, as Craig won't discharge you if you're sick. With a heavy heart but a grateful stomach, I dumped what chocolate was left in the open boxes in the trash and placed the remaining unopened boxes in all the visiting rooms and visiting areas on 3East, 3West, 2East and 2West.

Another temptation that came with my Independent Status was laziness. My laziness presented itself in the form of a power wheelchair. Using one of these, when you don't actually require the use of one, can lead to total inactivity if carried far enough.

I was given a power chair to test out about five days before going on Independent Living status and, since there was no immediate demand for such a chair, the OT department let me keep it in my room. Bad mistake! I calculated that by using the power chair I could spend a lot more time on my computer and then speed at full throttle toward any scheduled appointment and still arrive right on time. I would get funny looks from staff members and visitors as I zoomed past them. Hadn't I walked by them on crutches only minutes before?

Even more changes came with my new Independent Status. While I was snoozing on my couch after pool therapy, I was interrupted by my day shift nurse Shelbi. "Hi Herb, wake up," she said, "I'm here to teach you how to cath."

"I've been doing IC myself for over a week now."

"I know. You've been doing the "sterile method." I'm going to teach you the "clean method." "You'll use that from now on."

"*Oh Boy*," I thought, "*I just got comfortable and now it changes again.*"

I should have already learned by then that most abrupt changes at Craig were for the better. This was one of those changes. The sterile method of self-catheterization means just that. All supplies come in a sealed, sterile package: (Fig. 12–2) disposable plastic gloves, one catheter, one heavy plastic, sealed bag to attach the catheter to, one sterile towel to lay the supplies in, and three swabs containing an Iodine-like solution. In addition to the items in the Sterile Kit I also had four or five packets containing moist towelettes for cleaning.

The "clean method" required only a re-usable clean catheter. (Fig. 12–3) Instead of wearing sterile gloves you make sure you've washed your hands. In the sterile method the catheter empties into the bag and both the bag and catheter must be properly disposed of. In the clean method, you use the catheter in the restroom and let it empty directly into the toilet.

Since the catheters are re-usable they must be sterilized before the next use. Each catheter is thoroughly rinsed in very hot water immediately after its use. Then, just before going to sleep, you take the four or five catheters you used that day and soak them in a bowl containing a solution of water and bleach for ten minutes. Then you remove them from the bleach, rinse them thoroughly and put them on a clean surface to dry. In the morning you place them in a Zip Lock bag for use during the day. This method was simple to learn, easy to use and a definite improvement over the sterile method. Since there is no need to carry around Sterile Method Kits, mobility is greatly enhanced.

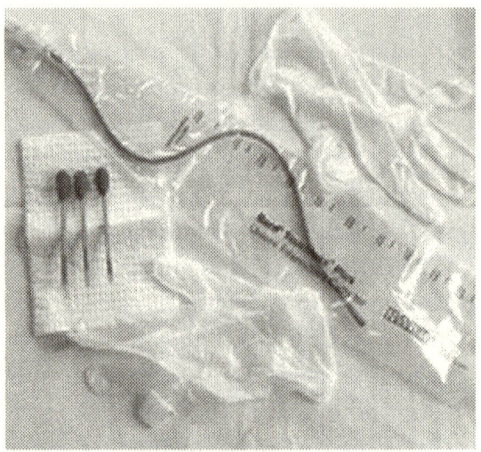

Sterile Method Items   Fig. 12–2

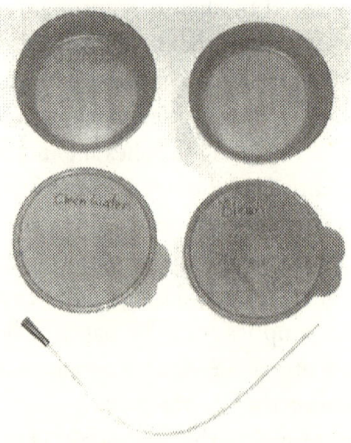

Clean Method Items   Fig. 12–3

Of course, not needing to use a catheter at all is every patient's desire and goal. They all diligently go through the muscle exercises they learned from their PT and OT to strengthen specific abdominal muscles and to keep others from atrophying or losing elasticity.

I tried hard in PT class to do exercises that would enable me to feel or at least control my bladder and/or sphincter muscles. The nurses encouraged me to try to void (urinate) without using a catheter, but I had no muscle feelings or normal urges telling me my bladder was full, so I stuck to my scheduled cath times. (I remained numb from my midsection down about six or seven inches.)

Around four-thirty the afternoon I officially went on Independent Living status, I decided (the one and only time) to take a little nap before dinner. I transferred from the wheelchair into my newly acquired double bed and closed my eyes for a nap. Then, after chilling out for ten minutes I suddenly felt an actual urge to empty my bladder. Thinking this was another false urge or spasm I didn't bother to get up. The urge got stronger so, putting my instincts aside, I sat up in bed, transferred to my power wheelchair and drove right into the bathroom where I stopped in front of the toilet.

Grabbing the handrails on both sides of the toilet, I pulled myself into a standing position and stood there, like I always did, waiting for the usual "nothing" to happen. I was prepared to stand there for a half hour if need be to see if the urgency feeling would dissipate. I stood there five minutes and was just about to leave when, without warning and without sensation, my bladder drained into the toilet. Wow!

I was so excited I didn't know what to do. I almost tried to run out of the restroom with my pants still down around my ankles but thought better of it. Looking up, I saw the cord attached to the nurses' station call box, and reached up and pulled it. The melodic voice of one of the unit secretaries, Barbara Ford or Cindy Hardinger, came floating through the speaker; "May I help you?"

Before I could answer her, my day shift nurse, Debbie Shultz, burst through the bathroom door. She'd been passing by my room and saw the emergency call light go on and, knowing that I wouldn't call unless it was urgent, rushed into the room to help me.

"What's wrong?" Debbie panted, still out of breath from running across the floor.

"I peed on my own!" I pointed to the toilet. Like a toddler being toilet trained, I just had to tell someone! Luckily, I'd avoided total embarrassment by having the sense to pull up my pants before she entered the room. Debbie started to laugh and then I started to laugh too. We both ended up sitting on the couch laughing.

Debbie explained that this was a good sign but it was probably a fluke. I'd still have to cath. She was right and self-catheterization continued during my stay at Craig. Many months later I had a chance to review my medical records and found a short note from Debbie that read: "2/20/05, voided for first time, 0500."

Another housekeeping chore necessitated by Independent Living was doing my laundry. My normal routine at Craig was to do my laundry only when I ran out of clean clothes, while others did their laundry at regularly scheduled intervals regardless of need. I kept my steadily growing pile of dirty laundry in a large, white laundry bag that I hung where I could easily reach it in the closet near my bed.

Knowing that I would be on Independent Status within a week, my OT Dana asked me whether I did my own laundry. Replying in the negative, I told her that Jill did it once in a while but usually the weekend techs took care of it, as the hospital was very quiet on Sundays. As a matter of fact, I didn't have a clue where the laundry room was. Dana knew exactly where it was—unfortunately.

Arriving at my door early the next morning, Dana picked up my laundry bag, dropped it in my lap as I sat in my wheelchair and said, "Let's go." I followed Dana down the hall past the nurses' station to a short corridor where we made a right turn and, Voila! There was a room with a washer, dryer and a long table to fold clothes on. *This'll be easy.*

Doing laundry was going to be easy if the washing machine was a front-loader. It wasn't. "Dana?" I asked, "How am I going to see into the washing machine when I can't get out of this wheelchair?"

"You're not," she replied, "Just roll the chair right up to the washer and I'll explain." Moving the chair against the washing machine, I leaned over and reached inside the machine. The washer was empty so I dumped my laundry into it, measured out soap, set the wash cycle, then Dana and I went back down the hall to the 3East lounge area.

Later and with little difficulty, I transferred my wet clothes into the front-loading dryer and went back to my room to wait for them to dry. While there, Dana went over the Craig laundry rules. The main rule, intended to avoid infections, was to sanitize the washer after using it, just as the person ahead of me had done. The next rule was really more of a hint than a rule. If I planned to do my laundry on Saturdays or Sundays, I should do it as early as possible. Patients' family members staying at the Family Housing Facility usually washed their laundry at 3East while they visited. If I arrived at the laundry room too late, the wait to use the machines could last for hours.

One of the advantages that came with Independent Living was the freedom to roam around the entire Craig Campus at will—whenever there was nothing else scheduled, of course. You had to check out with the duty nurse and get a pass if leaving the campus but doing this was a good idea so the staff knew where you were most of the time.

One day, when I had only six days left until my discharge, I decided to drive my power chair over to the 3West gym to use some of the exercise machines. I was getting a little nervous about leaving Craig and needed some physical activity to help me get my mind off things. I knew a little time using the wall weights and pulleys or practicing walking using the parallel bars would help immensely. (Fig. 9–4)

Wheeling into the gym I stopped by an elevated mat to heckle a fairly new patient, Dave Denniston, who was sitting on the edge of the mat using a large, brightly colored beach ball to play catch with his PT. This exercise is not about fun but about re-learning balance. I disliked it at the start of my rehab but came to enjoy it later. Dave, being an athlete himself, didn't seem to mind tossing the ball around at all. (*You can read Dave's story in Chapter 14*)

After chatting briefly with Dave, I went to the far side of the gym, and did some walking exercises using the parallel bars. As I was walking I couldn't help but chuckle to myself as I imagined what the atmosphere of Craig would have been like if Dave and Mark had been patients at the same time. They would have surely put Craig's socialization philosophy to the test. Both were funny, outgoing instigators and although I only had a chance to know them for only ten days each, they left a lasting positive impression on me. (However, I heard that some of the techs and nurses were relieved when they left Craig and the hospital was still standing.)

Independent Living required patients to accept responsibility for any trouble they stirred up. Sometimes this leads to situations where you wish you weren't so independent and had a tech around to help. The first night of my new status I got myself into one of these situations.

I had been signed off to shower myself without assistance and was looking forward to a nice hot shower to relax after a tiring day. Taking a shower requires advanced preparation, though. Although I could now stand myself, I couldn't walk without some kind of aid so I used my manual wheelchair to get around my bathroom.

My bathroom was large and the shower area easily accommodated a wheelchair except you don't shower in the wheelchair, you shower while sitting on a cushioned shower bench. The trick is placing the shower bench close enough to the shower knobs so you can sit on the bench and easily control the water flow and temperature. The showerhead is attached to a flexible metal tube so it can be removed from the wall and pointed anywhere.

The procedure for showering is:

- Wheel to the bench
- Transfer from the wheelchair to the bench
- Sit on the edge of the bench, steady yourself by holding on to a wall rail
- Push the wheelchair away from the shower area
- Close the curtain behind the wheelchair

If done right, you're left in the shower and the chair is outside of it, nice and dry.

Since I could stand, I found it easier to stand up from the chair, grab a wall rail then push the chair out of the way before I sat on the shower bench, which was placed over the floor drain.

The first night of my new status, I wheeled into the shower, followed the showering procedure, enjoyed my shower (using a lot of hot water while I was at it) then reversed the showering procedure. I pulled my chair into the shower and transferred from the bench to the chair. Then the trouble started.

Trying to wheel myself out of the shower and to the bathroom door, I couldn't manage to get any traction on the wet tile floor because of the steep uphill angle from the drain. The tires on the chair were smooth and flat and had no tread whatsoever.

I waited a few minutes then tried to move again. Same results.

I grabbed both of the chair's rear wheels and tried to pull my chair out of the shower, but that didn't work either. My only impact was to get the chair wheels sliding on top of the water. *I'm hydroplaning in a wheelchair?* If ever there was a time to panic and pull the emergency call cord, this was it, except, I couldn't reach it; it was on the opposite side of the bathroom.

For fifteen minutes I tried to get out of the shower but the floor just wouldn't cooperate. I decided I'd better sit back and wait for the floor to dry before I tried again.

Just as I was settling in the chair to make the wait a little more comfortable, my night nurse Kathy breezed into my room with my bedtime medications. She called for me.

"I'm kind of stuck in here, some help, please." I called out to her.

Kathy rescued me then but not before scolding me. "Not so independent yet?" she quipped, "Next time, use a long piece of twine to extend the cord on the call box so we'll know if you need help." *NOW you tell me.*

Independent "living" can have a lot of meanings but I found out first hand what the word *independent* really means. One February afternoon only five or six days before my discharge date, I was having an afternoon PT class with Heather in which I was practicing walking with only one forearm crutch. (Fig. 12–4) We were in the 3East lounge area where there were plenty of cushioned sofas and chairs and carpeting for me to fall on if necessary. I was wearing a chest belt as an added precaution.

I took only eight to ten small strides and then grabbed a chair or asked Heather for a crutch to steady myself with. I was ready to stop for the day. Heather saw this and said, "We are only twenty feet from your room. Why don't you try to walk there without any crutches? I'll be right behind you to hold the chest belt."

I needed time to digest her request. She was asking a great deal of me. After sitting on a sofa for a few minutes and enjoying some cold fountain water my evening tech Jennifer brought over, I thought, *"What the hell, if I fall it's pretty soft here."* *"Let's go for it,"* I said to Heather as I used the crutches and my leg strength to extricate myself from the sofa.

Standing, I handed both crutches to Heather and stared at my target destination—my bed only twenty long feet away. Heather put my crutches on the sofa and her hand on the back of my chest belt and said, "Just walk slowly and steadily. Go straight to the bed."

So, I did as she instructed and, sure enough, I was walking without crutches. I made it to the bed. Turning around to speak to Heather, I was stunned to find she wasn't there! She was standing back where I'd started, a big grin on her face. *That stinker!* After putting her hand in the chest belt, she'd let it slide out when I started to walk. Heather intentionally let me walk unaided, my first unassisted walking in ten weeks! I did it! I was *independent* again!

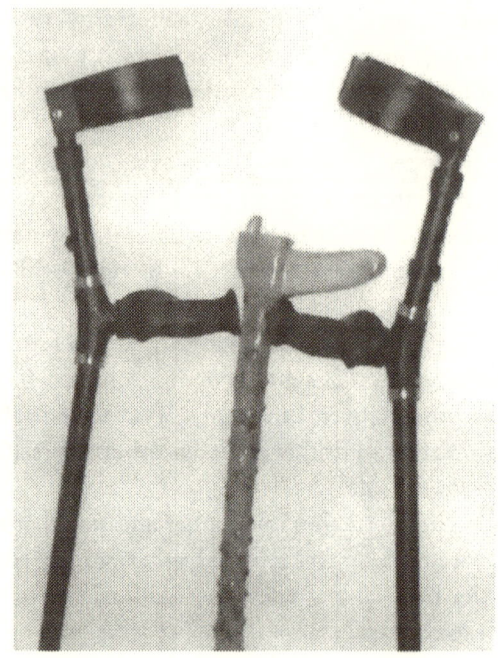

Cane and Forearm Crutches   Fig. 12–4

13

The Real World:
Facing the Future

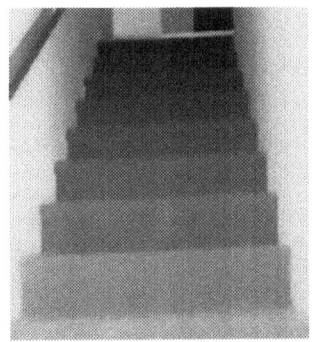

Fig. 13–1

When I was given a definite discharge date and went on Independent Living status, my stay at Craig was over. I certainly didn't feel prepared to leave the comforts and controlled atmosphere of Craig. *I'm not ready to be all alone. How will I get around? What if I fall and there's no one to help me?* With these questions nagging me, I tried, to no avail, to extend my stay at least another week.

While I could now walk a fair distance with forearm crutches or a walker and a shorter distance with a cane and could even take a few steps without any aid at all, I was still relying on my manual wheelchair for mobility. A few days before leaving Craig, I was summoned to the gym to be fitted for the wheelchair I would be taking home with me. This called for making some interesting decisions.

I had to consider circumstances I'd never even given a thought to. I was pummeled with questions. Was I going to be driving/riding in a large car, small car or SUV? Was the person who would be doing most of the driving able to disassemble, lift and reassemble a full frame chair? Did I plan to attend Craig's driving school to learn how to drive with hand controls and, if so, was I planning to re-equip my present car or purchase a new one?

"Hold on, everyone, one question at a time," I said. I sighed.

"OK, for at least the first month I'll be living with Michael and Jill" I told the OT, "Jill has a Passat wagon. She can't handle a full size chair." It just so happened, the only chair available was the smaller kind that folded by simply pulling the seat up. That answered the chair question.

I planned to attend Craig's Driving School as an outpatient but I was not making any decisions regarding hand controls until after I had a driving evaluation done. I intended to be able to drive before I left Craig but couldn't. In order to even be considered for driving training, every student must pass an eye test. I didn't even try to take the test knowing my eyes were still wacky from the steroids I was taking. Yet, one of the first things I did when notified of my discharge date was wheel down to the Driving School office to discuss the outpatient procedures.

Instructors Sue Phillips and Shad St. Louis gave me their business cards and told me Dr. Hsu had already medically cleared me to take the class. When I felt ready, I should schedule my eye test and other preliminary evaluations. Good, my first responsibility outside the hospital had been set up.

My second responsibility was arranging to feed myself and this meant going shopping, something I didn't like to do even before my SCI. The opportunity to test out my shopping skills came the Saturday before my discharge when Michael came to visit me by himself. Since I was cleared to leave Craig for short outings Michael and I decided to go have an Einstein's bagel and then head for the nearest supermarket.

After checking out at the nurses' station we went downstairs where I waited in my wheelchair for Michael to bring the car around. This trip gave us both an opportunity to practice what we expected would become routine. I transferred easily from the chair to the front seat of the car and Michael effortlessly folded up the chair and put it in the rear compartment of the car.

We drove to an Einstein Brother's store where I struggled while maneuvering the wheelchair through the door. But, after that, we enjoyed a fresh bagel and some coffee. We then found a Safeway store and, after unloading both the chair and me, we went in to shop. This turned out to be more difficult than I imagined it would be, as my prior weekday shopping experience with Dana had gone very well. Before, the store was fairly empty, but this time it was Saturday and it seemed everyone in Denver was there to shop.

Forget that I was in a wheelchair and probably deserved (and really expected) a little sympathy or maybe just some consideration, but what I got was absolute rudeness. Quite a few people shoved me out of the way to get to something on a shelf and others directed comments at me under their breath. Needless to say, Michael and I got out of the store as fast as we could.

Once back at Craig, I checked in and sank into the couch, worn out. The difficulties of the outing took me by surprise. But at the same time, I was very encouraged that I could handle the difficulties. I could take care of myself.

My next set of responsibilities was presented to me at my discharge conference the afternoon on the day before my discharge. I expected the usual attendees to be at the conference, with the exception of my PT Hugh who had left Craig the week before to take a position with a private rehab facility. Michael and Jill were there along with my sister Arlene who attended by telephone. Of course, being the guest of honor, I was expected to be there too. That was fine of course, but as a final display of the extent of my progress over my eight-week stay, I insisted I *walk* from my room to the conference room and back again.

The most direct route to the conference would be over the skybridge to 3 West and then down one never-ending hallway to the conference room. This would be, by far, my longest solo walk—no chair, crutches, walker or cane. Had I set too high a goal? I was going to find out.

Debbie Shultz, my day nurse and rehab team member, offered to walk with me to the conference and I accepted. I'm sure she had doubts about my ability to walk that far yet. I expected that talking to her would take my mind off the pain that walking produced.

We left ourselves a fifteen-minute cushion to cover a distance that Debbie normally covered in three or four minutes but Debbie didn't mind. I'll admit I had visions of collapsing just as I reached the conference room door. But nothing even close to that dramatic happened to me. Nothing happened at all.

With surprising ease and lack of pain and minus my usual muscle cramps, I took Debbie's arm and made my way to the conference room door. Once there, I released her arm to make the last five steps alone. As I entered the room, Dr. Hsu and all the other team members stood and applauded. I burst into tears as ten weeks of pent-up frustration, anger, pain, joy, sorrow, happiness and every emotion in between was suddenly released in one huge explosion. I was coming to grips with the fact that starting right there and then, I was basically on my own.

After a minute or two I regained my composure and the conference started. Dr. Hsu began by reviewing my rehab file beginning with my first day at Craig.

After that, each team member presented his or her final report and assessment. That was followed by what I'd been dreading, their prognosis and recommendations for adapting to living outside Craig.

Although my rehabilitation had progressed to the point of me being able to expend enough energy to force my body to walk short distances without any aids, my discharge diagnosis stated that I still had a long way to go before I reached anything near a full recovery. My medical diagnosis stated, among other things, "T-10 Paraplegia, Neurogenic Bowel and Bladder, ASIA impairment with profound Proprioceptive Sensation Impairment." (How's that for a mouthful?) In plain language the diagnosis said I was still paralyzed in a small area around my abdomen and had no feeling below my ankles.

The medical team members agreed with the therapy members that immediate and continuous outpatient care for me was not an issue. They also agreed I should stay with Jill and Michael in nearby Lone Tree rather than at the Craig Patient Housing Facility. My return to Breckenridge was unanimously voted down by every one present,—even by my sister Arlene over the phone. *"Oh well,"* I thought, *"Wait until I can drive!"*

After previously discussing the layout of Jill and Michael's house with OT and PT team members, it was decided I would occupy their guest bedroom on the lower level but shower in the bathroom on the main level.

The house could easily accommodate a wheelchair without having to construct any modifications, but we'd still need to obtain some adaptive equipment. Fortunately, my insurance covered the cost of the needed equipment that had been previously ordered. All I had to do was retrieve it from storage in Craig's basement.

As I said, my equipment costs were covered by insurance, but if they weren't, I would not have been denied equipment. This is because Craig has a policy: No patient leaves Craig without the necessary home equipment. This is made possible through the auspices and generosity of The Craig Hospital Foundation, a 501(c)(3) charity that maintains a Patient Assistance Fund specifically to provide this equipment for patients in need.

My final equipment list included:

- One easy folding collapsible manual wheelchair
- One cushioned commode seat (Fig. 13–2)
- One shower bench
- One set of toilet handrails

- Two slide boards, one short and one long
- Two reachers
- One pair of forearm crutches

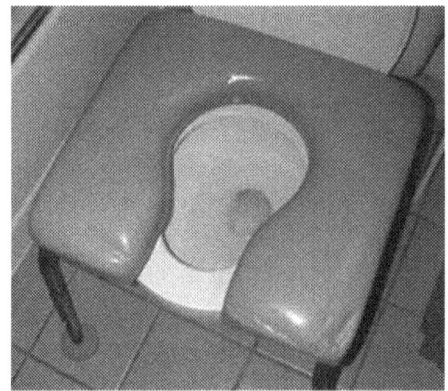

Commode Seat   Fig. 13–2

Added to the equipment list but actually given to me by Olivia was a walking cane carved of wood from a Florida palm tree.

In addition to this equipment, I left Craig with a seven-day supply of all my prescribed medication along with a written prescription for another thirty days and a red folder containing written instructions pertaining to all the medication. I also received a cardboard box marked "Supplies."

Inside the box I found a month's supply of catheters, examination gloves, and other non-prescription medication such as lubricants, skin cream, etc.

My discharge day arrived.—The morning I left Craig was joyous, sad and maybe even a little stressful. I was thrilled to be going to Jill and Michaels' house, saddened by leaving so many new friends behind and stressed by facing the realities that awaited me.

Fortunately my discharge was only from *in*patient care at Craig. My insurance company determined I was mostly independent and self-sufficient and therefore refused to approve any further inpatient care but the company acknowledged I was not totally able to care for myself. It agreed to continue coverage for *out*patient care at Craig. This was very important to me as it kept me in touch with the people at Craig and also gave me a chance to reach my goal of going back home to Breckenridge.

For the next three weeks, Jill drove me back to Craig at least twice a week to see Physical Therapist Beverly Parrott about my back pains. Beverly had been a physical therapist since 1966 and her firm, Physical Therapy & Injury Specialists, provided therapy services on 2East every Tuesday and Thursday. As my spinal nerves healed and I could feel some sensation again, my back pains increased and Beverly's therapy, along with the home exercise plan she gave me, were integral in keeping my rehab on course.

With my back pain now under control and my vision stabilized the one thing keeping me from re-entering a somewhat normal lifestyle was my inability to drive a vehicle myself. This kept me dependent on Jill and others to provide transportation.

Less than a week after leaving Craig, Sue Phillips, one of Craig's two Driving Rehabilitation Specialists called to remind me that Dr. Hsu had cleared me medically to enroll in the Adaptive Driving and Transportation Program. Although I was extremely happy to hear this, I knew enrollment was dependent on passing two prerequisites, an eye test and a clinical evaluation of my physical, visual, perceptual and cognitive skills. I made an appointment with Sue for the following Tuesday to take the eye test and evaluation. That gave me five days to vigorously continue my exercise program, eat a lot of carrots and worry I'd forgotten how to drive a car.

Tuesday came a lot faster than usual and Jill took me to Craig for an eleven o'clock appointment with my physical therapist Beverly Parrott which was going to be followed by my evaluation at the Adaptive Driving office. My session with Beverly was probably the best thing for me as her therapy session and the following few minutes of ultrasound treatment helped relax me and dissipate some of the tension I'd been building up.

After leaving Beverly, I went to 1East to the Adaptive Driving office. Both Sue Phillips and Shad St. Louis were there. I brought them up to date on my overall status and they gave me a now familiar stack of documents to read and sign. I scanned them fairly quickly knowing I had no choice but to sign if I wanted to drive. Sue then administered the eye test, given by putting your face up to a machine that had back lit numbers, letters and images very much like, if not identical to, the machine used at most state Motor Vehicle offices. Luckily, my eyes were pretty much in focus that day and I passed the eye test with relative ease. This qualified me to take the clinical evaluation test.

For obvious safety reasons, the clinical evaluation test was given on a computer driven simulator rather than in an actual vehicle. Sue pointed to a car steering wheel attached to a metal box on the edge of a desk then asked me to sit comfortably in front of it. This was the simulator. Sue adjusted my seat, the foot pedals and positioned the computer screen. "This is going to be just like an arcade game" I said to her, "But without the Dragons, I hope!"

Sue explained each test to me as it came up. All had one or—if needed—more practice sessions. Basically, I had to keep my car inside the lanes marked on the screen, while it moved at different rates of speed. Each test grew progressively more difficult than the previous one and included different speeds, more braking and in a few of the tests, faster braking.

Although driving started out as fun, by the time the last test rolled around I was sweating and had no idea how I was being scored. Using the simulator foot pedals was more than challenging, as I was still without sensory feeling in both feet. I was able to easily move them but could not feel them push on the pedals. This left me watching the screen to verify that I was braking properly.

When the final test was over I expectantly turned to Sue, but she just continued to write on her clipboard for a few minutes, completely ignoring me. Finally she looked up, smiled and said, "You scored better than a lot of Craig staff. Welcome to driving school. Now let's make an appointment for some road work."

We made an appointment for a couple of days later and I left the office to find Jill and get a ride back to her house. I could tell by the look on her face that she was not thrilled with the idea of me driving but she saw how happy I was, so I give her credit for saying nothing.

Two days later I was back at Craig and behind the wheel of a dual-control car. (A car equipped with both mechanical hand controls and standard foot controls.) Sue took me for an evaluation drive on the quiet streets behind the hospital which allowed me to get comfortable with the car and reacquainted with the feeling of driving.

In the next few weeks I would be working on my foot coordination with Shad and progressing from local streets to parking lots, to busier streets, lane changes and finally to interstate highways. This was a little intimidating but I was sure that Sue and Shad wouldn't let me try anything I wasn't ready for. Watching some of the other SCI students struggling just to get into a vehicle, I realized how fortunate I was.

What truly amazed me was how simple it was to use hand controls. I had an opportunity to observe a number of paraplegic students operating a car or van and they seemed to do it with ease. Once in a while from the window of my room I saw wheelchair drivers enter their vehicles in the parking lot and drive away like any other driver.

I also had the opportunity to inspect the latest in wheelchair van conversions and factory-manufactured vans designed for wheelchair operations. Once a week one or two local auto dealers brought wheelchair conversion vans to the East Parking Lot for inspection by potential patient users.

While these vans are not cheap, their utility makes them almost a necessity. Most conversion vans feature a hydraulic system that lifts patients into the van and allows them to secure their wheelchair as a passenger or driver or to transfer from the wheelchair to the car seat.

On March 31, I finished the driving course and received approval to resume driving my car. In five weeks since my inpatient discharge from Craig, I'd gone from using my wheelchair to two crutches to a single crutch and finally to a cane. Now I was driving on my own! My car had been parked at Jill's house for months and was just waiting to be packed for my trip back to Breckenridge.

Jill and Michael were glad I wanted to go home but they were wary of how I would handle the three flights of stairs in Breckenridge. They suggested a compromise. Instead of moving back right away, I'd go to Breckenridge with them for the weekend and, if everything went well, I would return on my own the following week. Deal!

As expected, I had absolutely no trouble on the stairs and so, after spending the weekend being closely scrutinized at every turn, I returned to Lone Tree for one more night. Then, I packed my car and headed back home...at last.

I unpacked only what I needed immediately and settled in to enjoy being alone in Breckenridge, finally returning home from a planned three day weekend, fourteen weeks later.

This was a lesson in adjustment. I had to come to grips with the fact that obvious deterioration of some of my physical abilities combined with the higher altitude (close to 10,000 feet) was going to cause me to get fatigued at a rapid rate. I couldn't run up three flights of stairs with my arms full of groceries like I used to, because, first of all, I couldn't physically do it, and second of all, even if I gave it a try, I'd probably pass out half way up.

These problems transformed me into an expert in logistics. I now had to carefully plan each trip up the stairs to maximize my load carrying capacity. I had to repack every bag of groceries from City Market in order to evenly distribute the weight, wear a jacket with deep pockets so I could stuff cans into them and I had to put items in a backpack.

Going to the Post Office the day after I got home also required some logistics. Breckenridge is still enjoying crowded ski lifts and lots of snow on its streets and sidewalks at the end of March. Driving to the Post Office in the snow would definitely be a breeze but getting out of the car and walking up the steps to the door would definitely be a problem. Still using at least one forearm crutch for dry pavement, I had no idea whether or not I would be able to walk in the snow. I sure didn't want to make an ass of myself by falling down in front of the crowd I imagined would be gathered there.

Breckenridge has lots of tourists but few permanent residents, so it is basically a small town. It has no mail delivery, so every individual, family and business must maintain a post office box. This is not as inconvenient as someone may think, reaching the Post Office from anywhere in Breckenridge only takes ten minutes at most.

Mainly, the Post Office is the unofficial meeting place, especially close to noon on weekdays.

At those times, you get to know many people, get many chances to talk to the mayor, town councilmen, county judges and any one else who might come in to get their mail. Congregating outside the Post Office was common so I felt some trepidation about trying to walk up the steps once I got there.

My worry was for nothing (of course). I found a parking spot right in front of the building and got out of the car slowly and carefully. The snow had been shoveled away so I decided to use one crutch and just go for it. I remember how slippery the packed snow was but I made it up the steps and down again without incident. This really boosted my confidence and allowed me to relax somewhat.

I drove back to my house, climbed the steps and, after throwing some small logs into the fireplace, lit a fire and just sunk into my favorite chair to relax. Aaahhhh. Sitting there by the fire, I had a chance to ponder my situation. I realized how much easier it had been for me to face the changes that were occurring than it was for some others I had met at Craig.

Hopefully, I was finished using my wheelchair although I had been advised to use it if my back continued to give me trouble. My only obvious problem was getting my balance steadied, which after I did, I had little trouble maintaining it.

I was also thankful I didn't have to undertake any house renovations other than repair my stairway railings that I needed for support. I thought of what modifications would have been required if I needed a wheelchair all the time, especially a power chair. Looking around my living room, the answer was obvious. None. I would have had to move to another house, as it would have been impossible to modify a three-story house into a one-story house.

Many of my fellow patients had to start adapting their homes soon after they were admitted to Craig. Jaime and the other patient counselors made sure that the patients and/or their families were aware of the importance of making sure that an acceptable environment awaited each patient when they were discharged. Craig could supply the necessary equipment but, with assistance from the Craig staff, the families had to ensure that home modifications were taken care of.

Home modifications could be simple or complex. In many instances, a supportive family, friends and others make constructing the modifications easier. My young friend Courtney lived on a small farm in rural Colorado. The entire town rallied around her after her injury. Several volunteers chipped in to build a wooden wheelchair ramp for her house so she could get in and out of it easier.

Drew, the attorney from Colorado Springs, orchestrated his home's modifications while he was in rehab at Craig Hospital. Family, friends and members of the El Paso County Bar Association assisted in replacing the carpeting with wooden flooring, making some room modifications and, thanks to having a high ceiling in the garage, raising the floor of the garage to eliminate the steps into the house.

I was sitting in my chair. I was home. Closing my eyes to better relax and soak up the warmth of the fire, I briefly forgot about myself and the many obstacles that surely remained to be overcome, and realized that facing the real world with SCI was unique to each person and handled uniquely by each person. The best I could do was to be as mentally and physically prepared as possible. Look out world!

14

Craig Grads & Patients:
A Few Stories

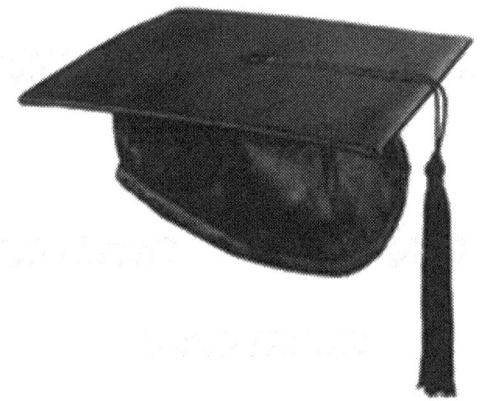

Fig. 14–1

One of the most gratifying things about my rehabilitation experience at Craig was the socialization among the patients. Constant interaction in the hallways, recreation areas, classrooms, cafeteria and everywhere else in and around the Craig campus was an encouraged, accepted, and welcome daily routine for me. After only a few days, my first name was well known, not only by the staff, but also by the patients. Everyone greeted everyone else in passing and even in the rehab gym. I often heard an encouraging "Good Job!" coming from fellow patients and staff just when I was struggling and needed it.

Patients were frank with each other about the nature of their injuries and openly discussed details of their accidents, rehab progress, and medical treatment. They discussed things they normally wouldn't have discussed with friends and family. (Sharing a commonality of SCI brings a camaraderie that is as strong as those found with college classmates, fraternities, sororities, and organized sports.)

In previous chapters I related incidents that occurred during my stay at Craig that involved fellow patients. To do justice to these patients and to pass on how well they have adapted to their individual situations, I am pleased to relate some of their stories and report on their progress as of this writing. I include each individual's website address (if available) where more current information about them can be obtained.

Dave

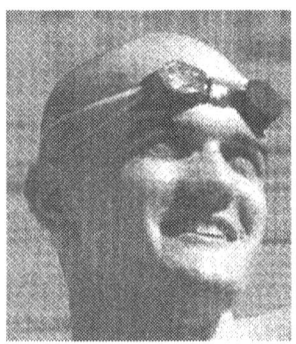

On February 6, 2005, Dave Denniston was spending some recreation time with a friend in the mountains near Laramie, Wyoming, his home state, sledding down the snow-covered slopes. On his last run, Dave slammed into a tree causing severe spinal damage and leaving him paralyzed below the waist. In addition, surgery was required to fuse his T-9, T-10, T-11 and T-12 vertebrae and remove bone chips. Dave remained in Poudre Valley Hospital in Fort Collins, Colorado for ten days after the surgery and then was moved to Craig Hospital to begin his SCI rehabilitation.

A 2002 graduate of Auburn University, Dave now faced physical challenges daunting even to him. During his years at Auburn as a member of the swim team, he was the Team Captain, an Olympic Trials finalist, 1999 NCAA Champion in the 200 meter breaststroke, and member of the 2003 U.S. World Championship Swim Team.

Dave's progress has been outstanding since his discharge from Craig. He has recently been able to stand and has some return of movement in his legs. Strongly supported by his many friends, family and Auburn University swimmers and Alumni, this year's Auburn swimming program Session V summer camp changed its name to the Dave Denniston Camp. For more information about Dave and to view many pictures, please visit his website: www.davedenniston.com.

Courtney

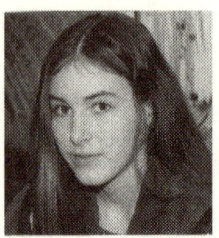

On October 27, 2004 Courtney Ferrall was riding in a truck with three of her friends, all senior classmates at North Park High School in Walden, Colorado. Heading to one of her friends' home to have lunch, the truck they were in suddenly spun out of control and rolled, four times, ejecting all the occupants. Two of Courtney's friends were killed instantly and the third died on the way to the hospital a short time later.

Still recovering from a spinal fusion operation only three months previously, Courtney was the weakest of the four before the accident but the only survivor. However, she was seriously injured and sustained a broken right leg, punctured lung and crushed vertebrae in her spine that resulted in paralysis below the waist. In addition, the nature of the injuries mandated immediate surgery to remove the hardware implanted during the previous spinal fusion operation. This was done at Children's Hospital in Denver and, after a week of post-op treatment, Courtney transferred to Craig Hospital in Englewood.

After undergoing the usual tests all new patients must do, Courtney was fitted for a wheelchair and started her rehabilitation program. Unfortunately, she was in so much pain that her program was severely curtailed and, after consulting with various specialists, she returned to Children's Hospital for another spinal fusion operation and repair of a new bone fracture. One week later, Courtney returned to Craig and started her rehab program again. This time she was able to benefit from all the hard work required to be successful and completed the program.

Her beautiful smile and positive attitude was an inspiration to the other Craig patients and her antics made everyone laugh—probably made the staff unhappy at times too. A few days before her scheduled discharge, Courtney's Mom, Millie, gave a big Thank You Party in the 3East lounge area. The party was great and the food terrific but it would have been better if Courtney had been there. She had stomach flu and spent the night of the party plus the next few days in her room.

Courtney has been living at home for over nine months, is doing great and recently returned to Craig as an outpatient for a scheduled re-evaluation. The entire population of the Northpark area has adopted her and many helped her adaptation by constructing a wheelchair ramp and other modifications for her home. Courtney graduated with her high school class and attended her Senior Prom. She was working in a restaurant and, as soon as hand controls can be installed in her truck, will be driving again.

To learn more about Courtney Ferrall and view more pictures go to her website: www.northpark.org/courtney

Drew

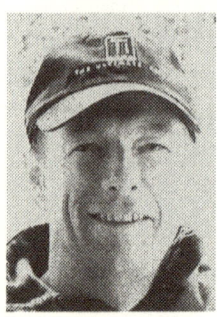

On December 30, 2004 Drew Wills was skiing with his family at Hylands Mountain in Aspen, Colorado. Drew, deciding to ski down the steep face of Garnish, failed to notice another skier traversing the hill right towards him. At the last moment, Drew saw the skier and, in a collision avoidance maneuver, made a quick cut to the right that caused him to lose a ski and sent him out of control towards a large tree. At the last second Drew twisted to avoid hitting the tree with his helmeted head but hit it with his lower back instead, crushing vertebrae and severing his spinal cord (T-12), leaving him paralyzed below the waist.

Drew had to undergo surgery to repair the crushed vertebrae and later developed some medical complications that prolonged his stay at Craig for a while. Drew and his wife Jeanie, with lots of help from family and friends, have taken their upbeat and positive attitude to an unusually high level of acceptance and adaptation. Drew is back in the courtroom as a practicing trial attorney and his house (including the garage) has been modified to make it wheelchair friendly.

In the summer of 2005, Drew (riding a recumbent bike) and Jeanie participated in a seven-day bicycling event held in the Colorado Rocky Mountains. Drew and Jeanie remain active at Craig through re-evaluations and their interest in the promises that Research may bring. Drew was interviewed for a short documentary highlighting Craig's fund raising efforts for research called "Push 2005—Stepping Into The Future."

More information about Drew can be found at: www.drewwills.com

Amanda

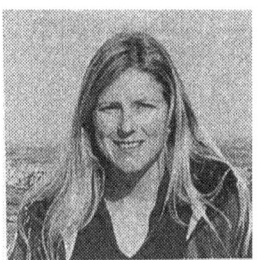

Amanda Vargo is a bicycle racer who was vacationing in North Carolina to relax after a race. On May 25, 2003, only one day after she'd completed the race, Amanda and her husband, Rob, decided to take a bike ride so Amanda could recover. Approaching a downhill curve at 32 to 36 miles an hour with Rob leading, two dogs ran into the road and blocked their path. Rob signaled Amanda to stop and she applied the brakes to her bike. Unfortunately, the front wheel brake locked causing Amanda to be launched from her bike, over the handlebars and onto the roadway where she landed on the back of her head and shoulder. Despite wearing a helmet, Amanda suffered a basal skull fracture and a broken collarbone.

The TBI from the injury left Amanda with moderate to severe amnesia and the inability to walk. After spending two and a half weeks as an inpatient at Craig followed by five weeks as an outpatient, Amanda overcame her dizziness, lack of depth perception and amnesia and is now fully recovered. In training again for racing, Amanda volunteers one day a week as an assistant to RPT Carol Aikin at Craig, giving aquatic therapy to TBI and SCI patients.

Earl

In early December 2004, Earl Rodriguez was driving on a logging road on his way home from work as a heavy equipment operator in rural Louisiana. Stopping his pick-up truck at the intersection of two heavily wooded logging roads he heard some popping sounds and then realized he had been shot. Within a few seconds, two teenage boys pulled open the truck door and took Earl's wallet. Unable to move his legs, Earl was helpless. Without saying a word, the boys ran off into the woods leaving Earl lying paralyzed on the front seat of the truck.

Using great ingenuity, Earl took a bucket that was on the floor of the truck and pushed down on the accelerator while steering with his left hand. He drove about a half mile to where the logging road left the woods and intersected with a highway. Once there he saw a school bus stopped only a few hundred feet away. Earl intentionally drove the truck into the ditch right in front of the bus. This got the bus driver's attention.

After running over to Earl, the driver called for assistance that came within a few minutes. It only took a few hours before the teenagers, ages 17 and 15, were apprehended and sent to jail where they still remain awaiting trial.

Earl has returned to his home in Louisiana where he gets around in a ¾ ton pick-up truck equipped with a swivel seat and hydraulic lift. His truck is fitted with hand controls and, Earl says that, except for the seat being a tad too high, he drives it without any problems.

Mark

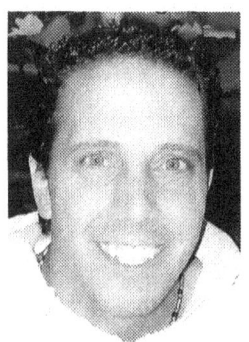

Sunday, November 7, 2004 found Mark and Alissa Gedman enjoying their first full day of vacation on a beach in Cancun, Mexico. Just prior to lunch, Mark wanted one more run in the waves so he handed his sunglasses to Alissa and took off towards the surf. A few moments later Alissa noticed what she thought looked like someone floating face down, snorkeling, but soon realized it was someone in trouble. Racing down to the water, she reached the person and, after turning him over, realized it was Mark. As Mark later recalled, he remembers body surfing into a wave when it crested and threw him head first into a sand bar. With help from bystanders, Mark was pulled onto the beach where he waited for an ambulance to arrive to take him to the hospital.

Hospital x-rays confirmed that Mark had suffered a C-5 level broken neck and had bone fragments in his spinal cord. Immediate surgery was required with his neurosurgeon using a piece of bone from Mark's hip to perform the required spinal fusion. After spending a few days recovering from the surgery, Mark was flown by air ambulance back to a hospital near his home in Boston where he stayed for a week before transferring to Craig Hospital to begin his rehabilitation.

Mark's progress at Craig was steady and positive as he progressed from quadriplegia to walking with forearm crutches, sometimes with great difficulty. With Alissa there to cheer him on, Mark became the "Energizer Bunny" of 3East, never stopping or slowing down, and setting an example for the other patients to follow.

Mark has been back home for nine months and has made considerable improvement although he still remains weak on his left side and had some problems with his left hand. Alissa and Mark recently returned to Cancun to revisit the site of his accident as well as to visit and thank the hospital staff for the care provided to him. Mark and Alissa keep an update and other information on their website that can be located at: www.markgedman.com

Kate

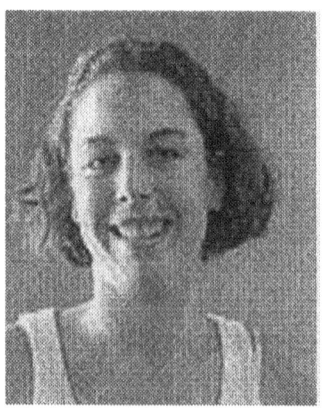

Kate Kimberly is a 2001 graduate of Colgate University with a degree in Geology and an obsession with western mountains. After college, Kate moved to Jackson Hole, Wyoming where she enjoyed the outdoor life, especially backcountry powder skiing. On March 20, 2003, Kate and some friends set out to find the Teton backcountry's last powder stashes of the season. After skiing the powder for a while, Kate dropped into a narrow chute but she missed her landing and lost a ski. Unable to maintain her balance, she skidded to the side and fell 240 feet off a rocky cliff, landing in soft snow but suffering a shattered spine and severed spinal cord.

Kate's initial rehab was at the Shepard Center in Atlanta, Georgia where she went to be close to her family. Determined to prove her doctors wrong about their stated slim chances for her independence, recovery and active sports participation, and also because she yearned for the mountains, Kate moved to Colorado and entered Craig's Outpatient program. Taking advantage of the opportunities at Craig and throughout Colorado and defying her original prognosis, Kate has skied, hand-cycled, rock climbed and even walked (with braces).

Encouraged by her own successes, Kate wanted to share her learning experiences with others in a similar situation. With the help and backing of family and friends, The Kate Kimberly Foundation was formed to help inspire, encourage and assist other people living with SCI and to raise money to help fund innovative research aimed at treating and curing SCI.

However, on March 22, 2005 Kate was severely injured in an automobile accident when the car in which she was a passenger rolled several times, pinning her inside. Despite suffering multiple fractures, Kate again refused to give up, is now well on the road to recovery and has returned to assisting others through the active management of The Foundation.

Information about Kate, the Kate Kimberly Foundation and the Kate Kimberly Foundation Annual Indoor Triathlon can be found at: www.katekimberly foundation.org.

15

Intangibles & Observations

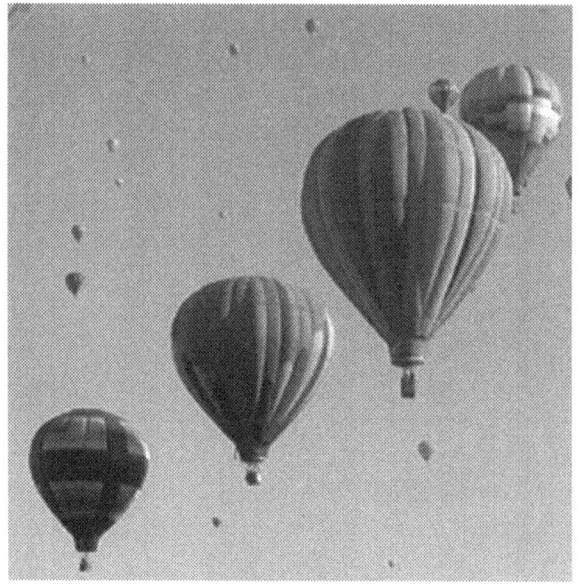

Fig. 15-1

The rehabilitation program at Craig Hospital recognizes that there are certain intangible factors that have strong influences on the progress of any patient. While there can be many intangibles for any one individual patient, every patient's rehabilitation success is directly affected by the three f's: Faith, Family and Friends.

A patient's faith in the rehab process is considered key to the entire program and is always being reinforced. Craig Hospital discovered a long time ago that mental determination went a lot further in fostering recovery than physical strength did.

There is no way to understate the importance of faith in achieving any positive result in the rehabilitation process. But exactly what is faith? Is it religious faith, family faith, faith in medical treatment, faith in you, or faith in community acceptance? The answer to this question is "all the above."

Religious faith is a nebulous factor that has a definite psychological bearing on rehabilitation. If you come from a strong religious background you definitely have a start in the right direction. SCI and TBI both have the affect of creating a need or desire to return to or embrace religion to discern why the injury happened.

Of course, a few patients angrily turn away from previously held religious beliefs to lay blame for their abrupt change of life. Also, what religion might be embraced to ensure a positive result? Should one choose Judaism, Christianity or Islam? If Judaism, should it be Orthodox, Conservative or Reform? If Christianity, should it be Catholic, Greek Orthodox, Methodist, Quaker, Latter Day Saints, or one of the many other options. This choice poses a problem for the patient and the patient's family but, in fact, the problem is minor. I feel that any religion is the correct choice, provided belief in its teachings is a catalyst to recovery. In other words, belief in the belief is the key.

The brain is the least understood organ in the human body, and mind is the least understood stimulus of the brain. The mind can make wondrous things happen that often defy scientific explanation. This truth has been repeatedly demonstrated in SCI rehabilitation.

Medical Science says SCI patients can never recover the abilities that are now considered reachable goals: A quadriplegic feeding himself, a paraplegic walking with the aid of crutches, another patient voiding on her own; these are results unheard of only a few years ago.

These accomplishments are possible because of a combination of factors. First, patients must have an unflagging faith that they will recover. Hope for the possibility of recovery is not good enough. Patients who show either the greatest recovery or the best adaptation in the community share a common link. They have strong faith in themselves, their religion and/or their rehabilitation program. The operative word is *faith*. Strong faith allows the body to heal and the stronger the faith the more demanding the mind is toward healing.

Craig Hospital encourages this kind of healing faith in two ways. First, it stands by its commitment to limit rehabilitation specialization to SCI and TBI patients only. This allows all of its resources to be dispensed toward rehabilitation benefits for every Craig patient. Second, Craig's environment is guided by its philosophy so the environment is set up to foster both faith and a positive attitude.

Planned socialization of patients with staff, combined with the emphasis on independent living, gives patients the opportunity to observe the other patients' progress and often gives them the needed impetus to work harder for rehabilitation than they might normally work. There's nothing like peer pressure to motivate someone to change, and the social environments at Craig definitely encourages forming peer connections.

Faith is reinforced at Craig in a variety of ways, some subtle and some outrageous. The subtle ways include making sure the staff is always positive with each patient and offer words of encouragement even when it is obvious the patient is struggling with a particular task.

I observed this subtle approach in action one day while on the mat in PT class in the 3West gym. A quadriplegic SCI patient, whose name I don't remember, was lying on his back on a mat having his legs exercised by his PT. He was trying to do an exercise that would allow him to move his upper body ever so slightly and was straining mightily just to get a muscle to twitch. He failed to accomplish the movement but his PT and others nearby came over and encouraged him with a couple of "Great tries" so that he kept trying until he found the strength in an arm to push slightly off the mat, the first arm movement he had since his injury.

Another subtle method used to bolster faith is the use of Craig grads and other spinal cord injured speakers to come to Craig to talk to the patients and their families. Being able to listen to the stories of overcoming adversity, watching videos of athletic achievements accomplished while disabled and seeing Craig staff in wheelchairs every day strongly reinforces a patient's faith in his own ability to recover.

From a patient's point of view, the speakers that were enthusiastically received were those that were enthusiastic themselves and related their own personal experiences. The self-confidence and desire that comes from watching and listening to a Craig graduate relate his/her every day triumphs and failures are immeasurable. Reading pamphlets and watching videos don't come close to having the impact that hearing an SCI survivor's story does.

One of the more outrageous ways to reinforce faith is to poke fun at yourself and your situation knowing that many others preceded you and succeeded while maintaining a positive outlook and a great sense of humor. Stories circulate among the patients, some true, others questionable, about serious situations turned comical by well adjusted wheelchair users with a sense of humor who have people hold doors open for them even though they're perfectly capable of opening doors themselves or how they get themselves into strange situations.

Despite some of the stories to the contrary, patients are taught not to be rude to well-meaning well-bodied people who somehow think that just because you're in a wheelchair that your mind, ears and mouth stop functioning properly. These are the people that come up to you on the street or in the supermarket, stick their face right next to your nose and in a loud, slow voice ask, "AND HOW ARE YOU TODAY, SIR?" As much as you want to play the game of acting dumb and coming back with a sarcastic retort, it is always proper (and wise) to answer politely and wheel away.

Almost as important as faith is the importance of family. Family support is so crucial to successful rehabilitation that Craig makes it as easy as possible for patients' family members to be with the patient whenever they desire. The new Patient & Family Housing building, located adjacent to Craig's East Building, contains apartments for families which Craig provides free of charge for the patient's first 30 days at Craig. When necessary, longer low-cost stays are arranged.

Taking another step to encourage family support, Craig has no formal visiting hours and allows visitors at any time as long as they don't disturb other patients. Family members and friends are not only encouraged to visit, but also encouraged to participate in the scheduled rehabilitation. The patient does not get excused from his scheduled class when a visitor is there and the visitor is encouraged to join the patient in whatever class he is scheduled for.

While family participation is a good idea, it certainly causes some interesting moments, as I found out. During my stay at Craig, I observed many patients' spouses, mothers, fathers, daughters, etc. accompanying them to each rehab class. Most of these family members, if not from Denver, were staying with the patient or in the Family Housing building and formed a sort of support group. Michael, Jill, Jeanie, Alissa, Millie, Alvin and many others were as much a part of each day as the OTs and PTs.

There were times, however, when there were minor conflicts. Once, as I related in a previous chapter, a few patients wanted to use the pool and brought the family with them, which made for a very crowded pool area. Some family members actually donned bathing suits and would go into the pool to assist with the therapy during scheduled class sessions. One of the couples that regularly shared this experience was Jeanie and Drew Wills who I would meet at the pool at least once or twice a week.

The other conflict came in using the laundry machines. I don't know what goes on that produces so much dirty laundry at Family Housing but for some reason, Saturday and Sunday early morning use of the washer and dryer on 3East seemed to be monopolized by Family Housing residents. Not that I minded waiting on line for the washer, but when other peoples' washed clothes piled up waiting for the dryer, I didn't like it because the chances of mixing up one person's clothing with another's, rose dramatically when there was a pile up.

Sometimes one family's show of support creates problems for other patients, visitors and Craig staff. For a few days about two weeks before I was discharged, a quadriplegic patient moved into the room next to mine accompanied by his wife and two children. The children looked to be about twelve and ten years old with the girl being the oldest and the boy the youngest.

While the family was officially staying at the Patient and Family apartments, they actually spent the entire day and evening with their father/husband. This is great if you are an adult but how do you keep two adolescents busy? Easy, you just let them fend for themselves and put them to bed when they get tired. How do two pre-teen children fend for themselves in a hospital? They play in the lounge area and race wheelchairs up and down the hallways.

At least the lounge area had tables and chairs where the little ones could sit and read, draw, paint or whatever. Racing the wheelchairs was another matter all together.

Taking advantage of the fact that no one was in the PT gym after six o'clock pm, the kids went to the wheelchair area of the gym where there were approximately 75 used manual and power wheelchairs waiting to be fitted for newly arrived patients. They each simply sat down in a manual chair and wheeled them back to 3East. There, they proceeded to race the chairs up and down the hallways ignoring the protests of patients in many of the rooms they passed.

Finally, some patients had been disturbed enough by the noise and dangerous use of the wheelchairs to ring for the duty nurse and activate the call button in their rooms.

The duty nurse that night was Lilia Smith who, most of the time was very quiet, but not this time. She happened to be in my room when the word came over the loudspeaker and she acted without hesitation. She opened my door and stepped out right in the middle of the hallway, put her hand up, and made the two racers stop.

"This is a hospital, not Disneyland, so act accordingly." She said just as she was starting towards the nurses' station. Lilia confiscated the wheelchairs and had them returned to the gym leaving the floor nice and quiet.

The families that learn every procedure that the patient learns are in much better position to assume the burden of responsibility and care upon the patient's discharge. Sometimes this learning is boring, dull and repetitive and sometimes it is fresh and exciting. I found some of the lectures extremely dull because I had no interest whatsoever in the subject matter being presented but some lectures were enervating.

One lecture I remember was one I attended with Jill. The subject was clinical research being done at Craig and was given by Dr. Daniel Lammertse, the hospital's Medical Director. The topic was fascinating and so was the lecture despite some technical jargon that I didn't quite understand. I got lost for a while and, judging by the number of quadriplegics sleeping in their tilted back wheelchairs, so did many others. The lecture did light a spark and I followed it up with many hours on the Internet looking up a variety of topics regarding SCI research.

When not attending class sessions or listening to speakers, most patients and their families enjoyed sharing new opportunities in Therapeutic Recreation (TR). Along with assisting a patient with crafts projects, the family members could enjoy the parakeet, watch movies on a large screen TV, plan for an outing or, when the weather was good, ride along with the patient and an instructor on recumbent bicycles. The TR department maintains a number of recumbent bikes that are driven while sitting horizontally to the ground with your legs out in front rather than the traditional bike where you sit on a seat with your legs going straight down. The bikes are powered by using foot pedals for able-bodied people and with hand cranks for paraplegics. Drew and Jeanie Wills took advantage of this opportunity and were often seen with their instructor, pedaling around the Craig Campus streets.

One of the most valuable intangibles that can occur is the ability to adjust to an SCI or TBI condition by discovering ways to re-focus that didn't exist prior to an injury. Many of us have talents or propensities that have been hidden inside ourselves and come to light only when exposed for the first time. The TR Department specializes in helping SCI and TBI patients and their families discover what talents lay under the surface that may be used by the patient to re-direct his energy from prior physical activities.

Being in a wheelchair doesn't preclude engaging in sports but discovering quiet activities brings relaxation. In addition to various types of artistic activities such as painting, sculpting, and ceramics, etc., TR offers pet therapy, music therapy and horticulture therapy. The greenhouse area of the TR department is filled with plants and it is not unusual to find a patient working there for hours.

In addition to the resident Parakeet, pet therapy is also provided through volunteers who bring their dogs to Craig one or two nights a week. When I was at Craig the dogs that visited in the evening were gigantic, hairy Newfoundlands. Despite their size, they were very docile and I liked playing with them. Their owners would come to 3East and just walk down the hallway and knock on your door asking, "Newfies tonight?"

Taking everything into consideration, my experiences at Craig were, and continue to be, exceptional and gratifying. While all of us feel depressed every now and then and wish our trauma had never occurred, we are grateful for each other and are sometimes quite surprised at our own ability to adjust and move forward.

Right after Hurricane Katrina devastated New Orleans and the surrounding areas I received a number of emails from Craig grads inquiring about my former roommate, Earl Rodriguez, who lives in Louisiana. I was unable to reach Earl until two weeks afterward and found out that he and his family had escaped the destruction but were without long distance telephone service.

Just the fact that people who had known us only for a short time took the opportunity to ask is the type of attitude that makes Craig so special.

Although my recovery is still ongoing and I have some bad days, I stay focused by keeping in touch with Craig Hospital, its staff and many Craig graduates.

Glossary

Catheter. A flexible tube inserted through the Urethra to drain the Bladder

Clean Method. Self-catheterization method using non-sterile equipment

Cystogram. Xray examination of the bladder

Cystoscopy. Examination of the inside of the bladder using a tube-like instrument similar to a catheter

Foley Catheter. Bladder draining catheter that remains in the bladder

Free Willy. Movie where a whale is placed in the water by using a sling

Googling. Using the search engine Google

Guillaume-Barre Syndrome. Neurological disorder usually resulting in paralysis from the neck down

Guldmann Lift. Electric patient lift using a jacket sling harness

Intubate. Inserting a tube into the Trachea for breathing

Lumbar Tap. Diagnostic procedure that drains spinal fluid

Moby Dick. The white whale in Herman Melville's novel of the same name

Murphy's Law. Whatever can go wrong will go wrong at the wrong time

Paralysis. Loss of nerve motor function

Paraplegic. Person with paralysis of the lower half of the body

Program. Self scheduled bowel movement procedure

Parkinson's Disease. Progressive neurological disorder causing limb weakness

Physiatrist. Physician specializing in physical rehabilitation

Quadriplegic. Person with paralysis of all 4 limbs

Reacher. Mechanical device to assist getting out of reach objects

Spinal Column. A series of bony structures (vertebrae) that hold and protect the spinal cord

Spinal Cord. A bundle of nerve fibers and cells that transmit two-way communications between the brain and body parts

Steinbrenner, George. Principal owner of the New York Yankees

Sterile Method. Self-catheterization method using sterilized equipment

Tech. Nursing assistant who performs medical and non-medical tasks supervised by a nurse

Tetraplegia. Same as quadriplegia

Therapeutic Recreation. Use of recreation services as treatment for persons with disabilities

Transverse Myelitis. Neurological disorder caused by inflammation across the spinal cord

Vertebrae. The bones that make up the spinal column

Yeager, Chuck. General (Ret) USAF, 1st man to break the sound barrier

Bibliography

Ayetey, Harold *Immunopathogenesis of Acute Transverse Myelitis,* 2002, Lippincott, Williams & Wilkins

British Brain and Spine Foundation *Transverse Myelitis,* 2000

Corbet, Barry *Spinal Network: The Total Wheelchair Resource Book,* 3rd Ed., 2002, Nine Lives Press, Inc.

Craig Hospital *Movin' On,* Fall 2004, Spring 2005, Fall 2005, Craig Hospital *Patient and Family Orientation Handbook Spinal Cord Injury Handbook,* 2003

Gerhart, Kenneth A. *Pathways to Health: You Do Have a Choice,* 2000, Craig Hospital

Kerr, Douglas *Current Therapy in Neurological Diseases,* 2001, Mosby Press *Immunopathogenesis of Acute Transverse Myelitis,* 2002, Lippincott, Williams & Wilkins

Levy, Charles *Transverse Myelitis: Medical and Rehabilitation Treatment,* 2004, Transverse Myelitis Association

Reis, Carlos Eduardo *Ataxia—Neurology,* Medstudentshomepage, www.medstudents.com

BluePrint for Health *Transverse Myelitis,* BlueCross BlueShield of Minnesota

Websites

www.craighospital.org

www.lifeonwheels.net

www.myelitis.org

www.spinalinjury.net

www.serenassong.com

www.bluecrossmn.com

www.medstudents.com

www.sci-recovery.org

www.med.umich.edu

About the Author

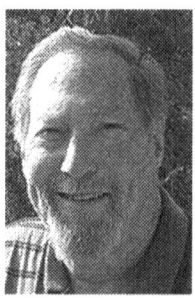

HERB TABAK

Herb spent most of his childhood on Long Island but will be visiting New Jersey this spring where he plans to join his classmates at Blair Academy to celebrate their 50th Reunion.

After a stint with the United States Air Force, where his Chinese language training was put to use in Texas, he received a Bachelor of Science Degree in Accounting from the Stern Business School of New York University, earned the Certified Public Accounting designation and eventually moved west where he practiced accounting and wrote numerous professional articles for national magazines and local newspapers. Along the way, Herb also earned MBA, JD and PhD degrees.

In addition to his accounting career, Herb is also a 2000+ hour Commercial Pilot with single and multi-engine, instrument and hot air balloon ratings. He is the author of numerous aviation articles and has covered the annual Albuquerque International Balloon Fiesta for local Colorado newspapers.

A regular contributor to the monthly *Cultural Times*, Herb is the author of *Where's the Runway? And Other Flying Stories* (iUniverse, 2001) and, with five other Colorado writers, co-authored *Colorado High Country Anthology* (iUniverse, 2004) a first place winner of USABooks.com BEST BOOKS 2005 competition and a third place winner in the Colorado Independent Publisher Association

2005 EVVY Awards. In addition, eight of Herb's aviation stories are included in *True Pilot Stories* (Infinity, 2005) a collection of stories edited by Patricia Lorenz.

No Whining is a true account of Herb's fight against Transverse Myelitis and his uplifting journey through Craig Hospital's unique and demanding spinal cord injury rehabilitation program.

For further information you can contact Herb at: writer756@earthlink.net

978-0-595-37814-2
0-595-37814-5